Praise for *Romancing Opiates:*

"In this thin volume, Dr. Dalrymple convincingly counters conventional wisdom regarding heroin addiction.... *Romancing Opiates* wittily argues that most beliefs regarding heroin are fictions, and furthermore that these fictions have had pernicious effects on both heroin users and societies in which they live."
  —*Dartmouth Review*

"In *Romancing Opiates*, a breezy, brave, and bracing assault on his own profession's pseudoscientific pretensions, Dalrymple concisely debunks the disease model of addiction ..."
  —Jacob Sullum, *National Review*

"From literary, medical, philosophical perspectives, he provocatively argues that uncritical acceptance of accounts of the nature of addiction has resulted in romanticization and misguided treatment efforts."
  —Booknews.com

"Former Birmingham prison doctor and psychiatrist Theodore Dalrymple has recently published *Romancing Opiates*: *Pharmacological Lies and the Addiction Bureaucracy,* in which he demolishes the medical model of substance misuse in the context of his description of a dominant Western liberal ideology."
  —Chris Byrne, *Mental Health Nursing*

"The importance of this book is not confined to shedding light on the myths surrounding drug addiction; it's a warning about what happens when an untruth prevails, and an examination of how 'where bureaucracies are concerned, nothing succeeds like failure.'"
  —Ron Smith, WBAL-AM 1090 Baltimore

Continued

"The book is eloquently written, weaving elements of history, literature, pharmacology, and personal philosophy into a plausible-sounding argument that may convince the reader with no prior knowledge of addiction."
—Roman D. Jovey, Medscape.com

"This is a hugely important book ... it could be a major landmark in the ongoing campaign to introduce truth ino the honesty-challenged issue of recreational drugs."
—Randal Cousins, lewrockwell.com

"Written by the witty and insightful British psychiatrist and columnist Theodore Dalrymple, this short, powerful book is one of the most important—and certainly one of the most entertaining—policy books of recent years."
—Betsey McCaughey of the Hudson Institute,
featured in the *Claremont Review of Books*

"Theodore Dalrymple has a knack for draining the fun and romance out of drug addiction."
—Christopher Orlet, *American Spectator* Online

"Dr. Dalrymple's experience as a prison doctor and psychiatrist in a large general hospital in a British slum backs his contentions: food for thought for any college-level health collection."
—The BookWatch, *Midwest Book Review*

ROMANCING OPIATES

Pharmacological Lies AND THE Addiction Bureaucracy

By Theodore Dalrymple

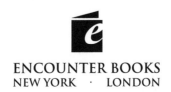

ENCOUNTER BOOKS
NEW YORK · LONDON

First edition published in 2006 by Encounter Books, an activity of Encounter for Culture and Education, Inc., a nonprofit, tax exempt corporation.

Encounter Books website address: www.encounterbooks.com

Manufactured in the United States and printed on acid-free paper.

The paper used in this publication meets the minimum requirements of ANSI/NISO Z39.48-1992 (R 1997)(*Permanence of Paper*).

Paperback edition ISBN 978-1-594032-25-7

The Library of Congress has cataloged the hardcover edition as follows:

Library of Congress Cataloging-in-Publication Data

Dalrymple, Theodore
    Romancing opiates: pharmacological lies and the addiction bureaucracy/Theodore Dalrymple
    p. cm.
    ISBN 1-59403-087-1
  1. Opium abuse—History.   2-. Medicine in Literature.
[DNLM: 1. Opioid-Related Disorders—history.   2. Fraud—
History   3. Medicine in Literature.
WM 284 D151r2006]   1. title.
RC568.O6D35 2006
362.29'3—dc22   2006004263

10 9 8 7 6 5 4 3 2 1

To Drs Sally Bradberry,
Robin Ferner & Allister Vale
&
The Staff of the West Midlands Poisons Unit

CONTENTS

PREFACE

In February, 2008, a man called Wright was convicted of having murdered five drug-addicted prostitutes in Ipswich, an otherwise unremarkable town northeast of London. The liberal British newspaper the *Guardian* described the five victims under the headline, "The women put into harm's way by drugs."

The father of one of the women said, "drugs took her away into her own secret world." The grandmother of a second said, "All she ever wanted was to be looking after her children, but heroin destroyed her life." The cousin of a third, whom the newspaper described as having taken heroin "for only a few years," described her transformation after taking heroin as "the flicking of a switch."

In the relationship of drugs to people, then, it is the drugs that should be deemed by readers to be the active party. Drugs are able—apparently without the intervention of human agency—to force themselves on unwilling victims, more or less as a tsunami overwhelms a coastline. It is as if drugs took people, rather than people took drugs.

This, I think it safe to say, is the predominant belief, both lay and medical, about drug addiction in general, and addiction to opiates (such as heroin) in particular. The belief is symptomatic of our infinite appetite for victims, no matter how willfully self-destructive they might be; for victim status is the condition upon which we extend our compassion. We are pitiless towards those who are responsible for their own situation; since we don't want to be pitiless, we deny the responsibility of those who, like drug addicts, make bad, and even very silly, choices.

Since the first edition of this book was published, I have seen neither an attempt to deny the elementary and publicly available facts upon which its argument is based, nor a refutation of its logic. A few of my own friends have dismissed what I say on the basis that it is absurdly right-wing. These friends assume that every argument about every subject can be neatly placed on a single political dimension, left to right, and that anything right of center is self-refuting. In fact, I cannot see that my argument is either left-wing or right-wing: I hope I shall not be accused of naivety when I say that I was merely aiming at what was the truth of this particular subject. If some people find what I say right-wing—tough. If others find it left-wing—likewise, tough. As the fictional English schoolboy, Billy Bunter, translated *Magna est veritas, et praevalebit*: Great is the truth, and it will prevail a bit.

At a public discussion of this book in Holland, I was accused of having set up a straw man. No one, I was assured by a professor of neuroscience, now believes in the propositions I am at such pains to expose as absurd—though, unfortunately, it is true that the very same propositions were believed only a few years ago. Indeed, these propositions still form the basis of public policy on this matter, which lags so lamentably behind neuropsychological enlightenment. No, says the Professor, we have now gone beyond all that, and reached the scientific truth, thanks to functional PET-scanners and the rest. We have proved that drugs alter neurology, brain cells, and neurotransmitters, and that therefore drug addicts cannot be held responsible for their own acts. Poor lambs, they need our help. If they don't get it, they are doomed to a life of everlasting torment.

And the latest (I feel almost tempted to say, fashionable) instrument of our sophisticated neuropsychologically-informed assistance to the victims of drug addiction? Motivational interviewing. What drug addicts need is a motive to give up. Hallelujah, I am also tempted to exclaim: and, exchanging dead languages for a moment, Q.E.D. as well. It was precisely my point that drug addicts needed reasons to give up, but that reasons belong to the language of meaning, purpose and intention, not to that of brute, physiological fact (except insofar as everything human belongs to brute, physiological fact).

If I am right about opiate addiction (and, of course, like all good intellectuals, I am open to correction), I illustrate in this book the baleful and philosophically primitive modern tendency to view social problems as merely technical ones, to be solved by narrowly technical means. This tendency in turn is a symptom of what my late friend, the great development economist, Peter Bauer, called the decline of connected thinking. Because of a surfeit of information, educated people find it harder and harder to connect disparate facts about the same subject, however obvious the connection might be.

The modern orthodoxy about drug addiction, I maintain, is not only wrong, but obviously wrong. As George Orwell said, "Sometimes the first duty of intelligent men is the restatement of the obvious."

INTRODUCTION

Men, it has been well said, think in herds; it will be seen that they go mad in herds, while they only recover their senses slowly, and one by one.

—Charles Mackay,
Memoirs of Extraordinary Popular Delusions and the Madness of Crowds

Man is the only creature capable of self-destruction, and only man decides in full consciousness to do what is bad, even fatal, for him. Freud's death wish may be mere speculation, an abstract construct conjured from the air, but no one with the slightest acquaintance with the human race could possibly conclude that human beings always pursue their own best interests by means of rational calculation. The primrose path to perdition never ceases to attract.

Not least among the attractions of the primrose path are drugs of abuse. This has always been so and will always be so. The temptation to obscure life's existential difficulties, dissatisfactions, and terrors by means of chemically-induced oblivion has always been, and will always be, great, at least until the meaning of life has been found once and for all. *Romancing Opiates* draws the appropriate conclusion from this: that addiction to opiates is a pretend rather than a real illness, treatment of which is pretend rather than real treatment. How and why addicts came to lie to doctors, how and why doctors came to return the compliment, and how and why society in general swallowed the lies wholesale, is explored in this book.

I

Not everyone yields to temptation, however, nor is the proportion of the population that does so constant in time or place. Our underlying anxieties about life may remain always the same (if this were not so, the literature of the past would hardly have any meaning for us), but our response to them is not always the same. It is affected by, among other things, the purpose that we choose to give our lives.

During the past fourteen years, I have worked as a doctor in a large general hospital in a British slum, and in the even larger prison next door. In that time, I have seen addiction to opiates—principally heroin—rise from an infrequently encountered problem to a mass phenomenon. Indeed, it has become so widespread that the city council has now put a request that citizens not put their used needles and syringes in the black plastic bags that it distributes to households for garbage collection. And no stairwell in a public housing project is quite complete without the discarded paraphernalia of intravenous drug abuse.

No doubt the sudden increase in the number of heroin abusers in my city was multifactorial, to use the word favored by epidemiologists when the proximate cause of a phenomenon is still unknown to them or anyone else. In all probability, the supply of heroin to the city became much greater and more secure, but no supply would or could have expanded so quickly unless it met its corresponding demand. The demand derived principally from disaffected adolescents and young adults who had been brought up to believe that the immediate satisfaction of personal desires was the highest, indeed the only, good, but whose economic prospects were, relatively speaking, grim, and who would never be able to fulfill their fantasies of a luxurious existence. Such young people were without the spiritual consolation of religion, or the distraction of a deep and satisfying culture. Reverie followed by oblivion was therefore their utopia. Even among young Britons of a higher social class and with better career prospects than the most typical drug addict, it is now common to hear the evening before extolled as a wonderful social event because the person extolling it was so drunk that he is now unable to remember anything whatever about it. This suggests a sub-Buddhist pessimism about the possibilities of human existence.

Before the sudden expansion of opiate addiction in my city, my acquaintance with the phenomenon was slight, and my interest less. I had known a few addicts in the higher echelons of society, but they had been self-evidently peculiar people even before they had started on their addiction careers. I had very briefly run a drug addiction clinic in a famous university town, at a time when I accepted uncritically what I now know to be myths about opiate addiction. As a person somewhat interested in literature, I had read De Quincey, but he had left little impression upon me apart from an aversion to overwrought prose styles. Opiate addiction seemed to me neither important nor interesting.

But as more and more addicts came to my attention—when I was on duty in the prison, I would see as many as twenty new cases a day—I began to think about it more. The medical perspective, which coincided with their own, that these people were ill and in need of treatment, seemed to me less and less satisfactory or convincing. The number of drug clinics in the city increased dramatically, as did the amount of medication prescribed to addicts, but far from getting better, the problem only worsened.

The condition in which the addicts arrived in the prison was pitiable. I had in my time traveled through many countries devastated by massacre and civil war, but still I was shocked by what I saw. At a time of economic prosperity, there were many young men who were quite literally on the edge of starvation. It would not be an exaggeration, but the plainest of plain description, to say that many of them looked as if they had just been liberated from a concentration camp. Hollow-chested and stick-limbed, they suffered also from vitamin deficiencies. Their tongues were the shiny smooth magenta purple of Vitamin B deficiency; the corners of their mouths were cracked. Their skins were pocked by sores. If any director wanted extras for a film about a concentration camp, he would need to look no further than the daily entrants to British prisons. I used to remark to such young men that if they were released from prison in the condition in which they entered it, everyone would conclude, and rightly, that we were running not a prison but a concentration camp. Therefore, I said, it was only reasonable to conclude that, for them, freedom was a concentration camp; their own desires acted as the concentration camp guards. Badly educated as they were, lacking almost all knowledge of history or interest in current affairs, not a single one of them ever failed to understand what I meant, and they always laughed; they agreed with what I said. Freedom was bad for them, because they did not know what to do with it.

In fact, the great majority of them stopped taking opiates in the prison, even when they were available. (They were smuggled in by various methods, the most unscrupulous and emblematic of which was the use of little packets of heroin placed in the rectums of babies brought on prison visits by the prisoners' girlfriends, and which would have killed the baby had they burst. In this milieu, of course, there are always other babies where, approximately, this one came from.)

The addicts came into the prison starving and miserable, and went out healthy and happy. Within a few months, however, many of them were back to their former condition, and not a few of them begged the courts, when brought once more before them, to imprison them rather than let them go free. A strange world indeed, in which incarceration is preferable to freedom!

When, soon after their arrival in the prison, I asked the addicts whether they intended to give up taking heroin, some of them would reply, "I'll have to, I've got no choice." I would then ask them why this was, to which they replied, "Because I've just had a baby and my girlfriend won't let me see it unless I do." In fact, this rarely led to prolonged abstinence, largely because the girlfriend in question soon found another boyfriend who objected to her continued contact with the father of her child. Most of the addicts emerged from a social world in which relationships between parents, between parents and their children, between children and their step-parents, between siblings and half-siblings, between boyfriend and girlfriend, between friends, between neighbours, were unstable and often violent, whether or not any of the parties was a drug addict.

Nevertheless, the answer given by the addicts—that the birth of their baby meant that they would have to give up taking opiates—was a strange one if they truly thought that they were ill and in need of treatment. They clearly believed that a purpose in life was a sufficient condition to enable them to abstain. This is not how pneumonia is cured. No one would say "I must stop having pleuritic pain each time I breathe deeply because I have just had a baby." The addicts themselves sometimes (not always by any means, for reasons that I shall explain later) acknowledged that their condition was a spiritual one, using the term "spiritual" in a loose sense, rather than a medical one.

I soon discovered that the medical services set up to assist addicts took a technocratic attitude towards them and their problems. They focused on the physiological aspects of opiate addiction, since these were susceptible, at least in theory, to medical intervention, which in practice meant the prescription of a drug rather like the one the addicts were addicted to. And there was a strenuous, almost outraged, rejection of the idea that addiction was, at bottom, a moral problem, or even that it raised any moral questions at all.

The addict was to be seen purely and simply as an ill person. And this meant that taking heroin was something that just happened to people, rather than something that they did. In the process of turning the addict into a blameless patient, therefore, the doctors, nurses, psychologists, counselors, and social workers also turned an addict into something less than a fully responsible person, into someone not in charge of his own behavior, a creature or automaton effectively without choices, intentions, or even weaknesses. So uncertain of their own benevolence were these functionaries of care that they avoided all mention of the moral and spiritual aspects of addiction, since even to mention them *en passant* was to risk being perceived as condemnatory and therefore malevolent in intent. In this odd little sub-culture (which nevertheless echoes prevalent attitudes outside itself) only those who approve of, or at least do not express disapproval of, other people's behavior can consider themselves or be considered by others to be generous-minded.

Of course, it cannot be denied that opiate addiction has medical consequences, many of them very serious. For example, I would often see addicts on their arrival in prison who had had deep vein thromboses or pulmonary emboli. When they arrived, they would often have multiple abscesses; they would have tuberculosis because of the way they lived; they would be malnourished; they would be infected with Hepatitis B or C, or both, and HIV; they would even have severe injuries for which they had sought no treatment. It would be difficult to obtain blood from the veins in their arms or legs for necessary tests because they had injected into them so many times that the veins had turned hard as cords; they would have injection sites in the backs of their hands, in their groins, and in their necks. A man who injects himself in the external jugular vein is unlikely to be much concerned for his own good health. I have even known of addicts inject themselves in the eyes and blind themselves rather than go without their drug, an act so horrible that the mind of a normal person turns instinctively away from it and cannot keep it long in consciousness.

But medical consequences, however terrible, do not make a disease. Many mountaineers break their legs or get frostbite, but mountaineering is not a disease. Sport is now one of the principal causes of injuries in the western world, but, however fatuous a sport may be, it is not a disease. And to conceive of opiate addiction as a disease seems, after my experience with thousands of drug addicts, to me to miss the fundamental point about it: that it is a moral or spiritual condition that will never yield to medical treatment, so called. Having myself started with a vague supposition that the medical approach to addiction must be right and compassionate, because that was what I had been taught by people whom I respected, I came by degrees to a very different conclusion: that such an approach, having started no doubt as an honest attempt to help addicts, now represented a combination of moral cowardice, displacement activity, and employment opportunity. In a modern bureaucratic society, after all, few are the social problems that cannot be turned to professional or personal advantage.

But the therapeutic juggernaut rolled, and continues to roll, on, the only explanation for its lack of success being that it is still of insufficient size. If only it were half as big again, or twice as big, or four times as big: then the problem would be defeated. Strangely enough, those in charge of the purse-strings have been only too ready to believe it, and have paid for a constant expansion. It is easier, after all, to give people a dose of medicine than to give them a reason for living. That is something the patient must minister to himself.

I began to feel that I was living in a strange world, one in which the plainest of truths before one's nose could neither be said out loud nor in any way acknowledged. It therefore seemed to partake of the atmosphere of Kafka. Every day I saw addicts who abused their prescription drugs from the clinics that were set up to help them, who sold them to third parties or who continued to take heroin, and every other illicit drug they could get hold of, in spite of and in addition to these prescription drugs; addicts who, despite their so-called treatment, continued to commit crimes; addicts who were openly contemptuous of all attempts to help them, and who lied to and manipulated their supposed helpers in a shameless and unmistakable fashion; addicts who had, without any assistance whatsoever, and without difficulty, abjured their habit completely; addicts whose histrionics were obviously and demonstrably dishonest; and above all, I observed close up the triviality of withdrawal symptoms from opiates. Yet none of my observations seemed to count for anything. It was almost impolite, and increasingly impolitic, to mention them to my colleagues who dealt with drug addicts, though they must have observed the same things themselves even more often. I felt increasingly not like a doctor whose clinical experience might be valuable, the starting point of reflection and debate, but like a heretic who had better keep his beliefs to himself for fear of drawing the institutional wrath of orthodoxy down on himself and making himself the object of an inquisition. Had I not been fortunate enough to work with three eminent and highly competent physicians in my hospital who had observed precisely what I had observed, and drawn the same conclusions, I think I might have broken down, for as every political propagandist knows, there is nothing more destructive of the human psyche than to be forced to doubt the veracity of what one's own elementary observations demonstrate, simply because they conflict with a prevailing and unassailable orthodoxy. In such circumstances, one is forced to choose between considering oneself deluded, or the world as mad: one is either sane in an insane world, or insane in a sane world. Neither alternative is entirely satisfactory.

I decided to give form to my growing dissent from the orthodoxy that had become the doctrine not just of the medical profession, but of the government and (insofar as it had any opinion on the matter) the population itself. How and why had doubtful propositions—no, manifest untruths—become so widely, almost universally, accepted, especially in an age that prided itself on its skepticism and unwillingness to take anything on trust? Why were the most elementary truths disregarded entirely, and no conclusions whatever drawn from them?

I grant, of course, that opiate addiction is by no means the largest or gravest problem faced by our society, that at some point its spread will cease, and that it will never seize hold of more than a fraction of the population. It might even recede somewhat. But if our society cannot even think clearly, honestly, and courageously, without deception or self-deception, about a minor social problem, what hope is there that it will confront larger problems clearly, honestly, and courageously? *Romancing Opiates* seeks to expose the willful misconceptions, the lies and evasions, of the past two hundred years with regard to opiate addiction. This, then, is a case study; it is a warning of what happens when untruth prevails; and it is also my personal exorcism or catharsis, after living for so many years in an atmosphere of lies, half-truths, and unmentionable facts about something that was essentially as plain as the hand before my face.

The history of the discovery of truth is important; but the history of the perpetuation of error is just as instructive in its own way.

I

Lies! Lies! Lies!

... upon all that has been hitherto written on the subject of opium ... I have but one emphatic criticism to pronounce—Lies! lies! lies!

—Thomas De Quincey
Confessions of an English Opium-Eater (1822)

The Misconception of the Problem

Heroin is the opium of the people.

If we replace "religion" by "heroin" in the famous passage from Marx's *Contribution to the Critique of Hegel's Philosophy of Right,* published in 1844, this is what we get:

> Heroin is the sigh of the oppressed, the heart of a heartless world, the soul of soulless conditions.... The abolition of heroin as the illusory happiness of the people is the demand for their real happiness. To call on them to give up their illusions about their condition is to call on them to give up a condition that requires illusions. The criticism of heroin is, therefore, in embryo, the criticism of that vale of tears of which heroin is the halo.

Our subject, therefore, though insignificant in the statistical sense, is a philosophically pregnant one.

Unfortunately, it is not only those who take heroin who are blinded by illusions, but almost the entire population, including—or especially—the experts. Every problem in contemporary society calls forth its equal and supposedly opposite bureaucracy.

The ostensible purpose of this bureaucracy is to solve that problem. But the bureaucracy quickly develops a survival instinct and so no more wishes the problem to disappear altogether than the lion wishes to kill all the gazelle in the bush and leave itself with no food for the future. In short, the bureaucracy of drug addiction needs drug addicts far more than drugs addicts need the bureaucracy of drug addiction.

Thanks to propaganda assiduously spread for many years by everyone who has concerned himself with the subject, there is now a standard or received view of heroin addiction that is almost universally accepted by the general public, by the addicts themselves, and by the bureaucracy alike. This view serves the interests both of the addicts who wish to continue their habit while placing the blame elsewhere, and the bureaucracy that wishes to continue in employment, preferably forever and at higher rates of pay.

This standard or received view conceives opiate addiction as an illness and therefore implies that there is a bona fide medical solution to it. When all the proposed "cures" fail to work, as they usually do, and when the extension of quasi-medical services to addicts is accompanied not by a decline in the prevalence of the problem but, on the contrary, by an increase, who can blame addicts if, in continuing their habit, they blame not themselves but the incompetence of those who have set themselves up as their medical saviors and offered them solutions that do not work? I wish I had a dollar for every addict who said to me that he would have given up the drug "if only I got the help." Of course, even when he does get the "help," he doesn't get the help in the sense that he necessarily and automatically gives up as a result of having done so, as a person with pneumococcal pneumonia gets better when he receives the right antibiotics: and he therefore concludes that he has got the wrong kind of help, which is what he both hoped for and knew in advance of seeking the supposed "help."

But where bureaucracies are concerned, nothing succeeds like failure. For example, the budget for the National Institute of Drug Abuse increased by 16.2 percent from 2001 to 2002 alone, which would be quite a creditable performance if it had been a purely commercial enterprise. $126,394,000 was added to its budget in the period, but it would be a brave or foolhardy man who asserted that a single drug addict stopped, or ever will stop, taking drugs because of this extra funding. Nor would you have to be Nostradamus to predict that the budget will keep growing, however many or few drug addicts there are, unless of course there is a general economic collapse necessitating drastic budgetary retrenchment. What one can say with a fair degree of certainty is that the funding of the NIDA will remain sturdily independent of the importance or usefulness of its findings, and of the social importance or otherwise of the problem it addresses. The bureaucratic solution to waste is always more waste.

It is true, of course, that the official bureaucracy of drug-addiction is a very minor partner of the drug-smuggling and distribution industry, with only a fraction of its resources, but it does have the inestimable advantage of being wholly legal and aboveboard. When it comes to honesty, however, it is a close-run thing. It seems to me likely that, from the standpoint of self-awareness, the drug smugglers are superior to their bureaucratic counterparts. Necessity is the mother if not of all, then at least of a great deal of intellectual honesty, and drug smugglers can afford no illusions. By contrast, illusions are a precondition of the bureaucracy's growth and continued existence.

The Standard or Orthodox View

The standard or orthodox view of heroin addiction is as follows, a view that—as we shall see—has a different function in the case of addicts, doctors, and the general public. According to this view, a man is somehow or other exposed to heroin, more or less by chance. It has a pleasurable effect on him, and he takes some more, and then some more again. Before long, indeed very quickly, he is physiologically addicted, and in order to avoid the terrible suffering caused by withdrawal, he has to take more and more heroin. Unfortunately, in order to pay for this, he often has to resort to crime, unless he belongs to that small elite of addicts who come from the moneyed classes, for his addiction precludes normal paid work but requires a large income. His powers of self-control have by now been completely destroyed or subverted by heroin. Unless he takes a substitute drug, or possibly enters a lengthy and technically rigorous rehabilitation programme, he cannot give up. He is hooked, and hooked for life. He needs help.

There is only a very tiny grain of truth in all this. That physiological addiction exists is undoubted. But in practically all other respects, the standard view is wrong. It is a masterpiece of the old rhetorical tricks of *suppressio veri* and *suggestio falsi*. It overlooks the most obvious salient facts. It is to heroin addicts what Marxism was to members of the Politburo of the former Soviet Union: a systematic pseudo-scientific justification for everything that they do, if not in their own interest, then in accord with their desires.

Let us take the standard view point by point.

The Beginning of Addiction

A man is somehow or other exposed to heroin. But how is a man exposed to heroin? The use of the passive voice is here very instructive. The heroin comes to the man, the man does not go to the heroin. It is as if the heroin had a will of its own, unlike the man. The heroin is active, the man passive. A fine, and not untypical, example of this kind of thinking came my way recently in the statement of a young criminal, charged with robbery, on whom I prepared a medical report at the request of his lawyer:

> When we moved to D_____, I just fell into taking drugs by the usual route. I met two blokes who were somewhat older than me and it all started off with a few drinks and one day one of them had a cannabis joint, I smoked that, things progressed, then on another day somebody brought in some crack cocaine, that was smoked and one thing led to another and then I find myself a heroin addict.

On this highly selective account, almost no human agency, at least on the part of the addict, is admitted. "It" starts off, "things" lead to one another, and a person finds himself in a position as if he had been kidnapped and taken blindfold by main force to a completely unknown destination.

Clearly, such an account is self-serving, in the sense that it implies no control, and therefore no blame. What, perhaps, is more surprising is that large numbers of well-trained, or at least indoctrinated, people—doctors, therapists, social workers, and the like—swallow such clearly self-serving accounts more or less whole. For reasons that I shall later hint at, they delight to view people with unfortunate backgrounds as being wholly the victims of those backgrounds.

But people who are genuinely exposed to strong opiates by chance, in medical circumstances, for example after an operation, in fact very seldom become addicted to them. The great majority of heroin addicts do not become addicted via the medical route. In fact, I do not recall one among the many hundreds whom I have met.

It might once have been the case, I suppose, before awareness of the addictive and other properties of heroin was so general, that unsuspecting persons were introduced to the habit by people who did not tell them of the habit-forming propensities of the drug, and who were thus "hooked" (another expression indicative of passivity, which reduces people to the moral and intellectual level of fish) before they knew what was happening.

But whatever may have been the case in the past, this is not a plausible explanation of what happens now. The great majority of heroin addicts whom I see in my practice—who are not untypical of inner city heroin addicts, and who are themselves the great majority of heroin addicts—come from areas of the city in which it is impossible to remain ignorant of what might be called the heroin way of life. Not only has this way of life been widely, if not always honestly or accurately, portrayed in books, plays, and films, but it is also on view to everyone from an early age. Children may not know any longer the dates of the Battle of Hastings or the Declaration of Independence, but they know that heroin is addictive and what kind of people take it. Many addicts say that they did not know what they were getting themselves into when first they took heroin, but this is simply not credible; they could not have failed to know.

When I ask heroin addicts why they started taking heroin, the great majority of them reply with one of two answers. These are: "I fell in with the wrong crowd," and "Heroin's everywhere." Once again, the addict is the passive partner in the relationship between heroin or its peddlers, and the addict. To fall is to be subject to the force of gravity, which it is vain for the individual to oppose. It is thus as impossible and fruitless to resist the influence of the wrong crowd as that of the force of gravity. And heroin being everywhere, it is as impossible not to smoke or inject it as it is not to speak one's native tongue or breathe the gaseous atmosphere in which one lives.

"I fell in with the wrong crowd." When I reply that it is odd how I meet many people who fell in with the wrong crowd, but I never under any circumstances meet any member of the wrong crowd itself, who must therefore be lurking permanently out of my sight and hearing, the addict who has attributed his addiction to his fortuitous acquaintance with the wrong crowd smiles, or even laughs, knowingly. Though usually neither highly intelligent nor well-educated, he knows exactly what I mean, and what point I am trying to make. A man who says that he is easily led (a second-order excuse of those who fell in with the wrong crowd) never uses this characteristic to explain his good deeds, good characteristics, or positive achievements. A man never claims to have been easily led to higher mathematics, the subjunctives of foreign languages, or unpaid work among the poor. People are influenced by the people they admire and wish to emulate: the admiration and the desire for emulation precede the influence.

Although I have known of cases in which heroin was administered forcibly to an unwilling person, they are very few. Not very long ago, a few hundred yards from where I write this, the body of a sixteen-year-old girl was found dumped near a reservoir. Two pimps had been trying to get her addicted to heroin in order that she would thenceforth work for them to earn the price of her heroin, and had been over-zealous in the quantities that they had injected her with, and she died. The girl, it turned out, was from a respectable middle-class family that lived in a small town nearby. She had run away from home, attracted by the glamour, as she thought it, of low-life in the slums of the city. She actually wanted to be a drug-addicted prostitute, rather than a schoolgirl whose exams were approaching. While her meeting with the two pimps could no doubt have been characterized as chance, it was no accident, as the Marxists used to say, that it was she rather than another girl in her class at school who ended up decomposing in the bushes by the reservoir. If she was a victim, she was almost as much a victim of ideas and images frivolously propagated by magazines and advertisers as of the two pimps themselves. It was during the vogue of heroin chic that she died, heroin chic being the latest manifestation of the ludicrous but recurrent notion that there is something profound, attractive, and tragic in the heroin or opiate-addicted way of life. The sullenly vacant expression of half-starved models was supposed to hint obliquely that there were matters on their minds deeper than mere clothes, as if intellectual profundity were merely a question of adopting the right facial expression and posture.

Nevertheless, falling in with the wrong crowd as an explanation of misconduct has a superficial plausibility. I have heard it many times offered, with every appearance of conviction, by the parents, social workers, and doctors of drug addicts as an explanation of why a young man became an addict. The wisdom of ages, that birds of a feather flock together, is simply ignored.

"Heroin's everywhere" is an alternative explanation. The addict means by this that it is inescapable; once again, the heroin comes to him, or even forces itself upon him, and hence there is nothing he could have done (or could now do) to avoid it.

But if heroin is everywhere, I ask, why is everyone not a heroin addict? If heroin is everywhere, it is everywhere for everyone. But the figures are quite clear: heroin addiction, however much it might have spread in the last few years, is still the affliction of a small minority, even in the worst areas of the worst cities.

Of course, it is perfectly possible, likely even, that people live in social micro-climates, in some of which heroin addiction is very much more common than in others. But there is no micro-climate, other than the self-constituted one in which addicts live, in which heroin addiction is absolutely universal, literally inescapable as it would have to be for its ubiquity to count as the explanation of any individual addict's addiction.

A person's initial consumption of heroin is not the result of a reflex, or of an irresistible impulse. No doubt there is often social pressure exerted upon the weak and vacillating to try the drug, to be real men or adults, to prove their daring by doing something that is forbidden, and so forth. No doubt this is also the origin of many a criminal career. But there still remains a choice in the matter: even where a certain type of misconduct is common, it is never absolutely universal. Second, even if undesirable social pressure of this kind were an explanation of the initiation of addiction, it would not be amenable to medical intervention. If an increase in the number of heroin addicts such as Britain has experienced in the last few decades—up from a very few in the 1950s (there were only 62 known cases in Britain in 1958, 670 in 1968, and as late as 1978 there were only 859, when heroin addicts were still few enough to be registered individually by the Home Office, which no doubt underestimated the numbers, but not by orders of magnitude) to well over 100,000 by the year 2000—constitutes an epidemic, it is an epidemic of a very strange kind, one that is spread by the psychological contagion of bad ideas and bad desires rather than by the physical contagion of bad germs. As for health education, which is supposed to be to drug addiction and other bad habits what vaccination is to smallpox, it does not seem to work. This is because knowledge is a determinant of human conduct only to a very limited extent, a determinant that is probably strongest among those with the least inclination to the supposed enchantment of opiates in the first place. The decline in cigarette smoking consequent upon the dissemination of information about its noxiousness to health has been greatest in the richest and best-educated portion of society, and least in the poorest and worst-educated portion.

The Addictive Nature of Opiates

On the standard view, opiates are highly addictive. The process of becoming addicted, if not quite instantaneous, is at least very swift. The public still believes what Ellen N. La Motte wrote in 1920, in her little book *The Opium Monopoly:* "after a dose or two the fatal habit would be formed." Having fallen into the wrong crowd, or having lived in a heroin-impregnated atmosphere, the future addict has to take the drug only a couple of times and then—hey presto!—his willpower is gone, like ice in a warm drink. He is hooked, once and for all, more exhausted fish flapping weakly at the end of a line than man. He is no longer fully in control of himself. He is like a Haitian zombie, a zombie whose actions are determined by heroin or by his supplier of heroin.

This is the sheerest nonsense. Actually, you have to work quite hard to become a bona fide heroin addict; indeed, there are many careers entry into which is far less exacting. De Quincey, in his *Confessions of an English Opium-Eater,* first published in book form in 1822, tells us that he took opium on Saturdays alone for many years before becoming an addict. De Quincey says:

> Courteous, and I hope indulgent reader, having accompanied me thus far, now let me request you to move onward for about eight years; that is to say, from 1804 (when I said that my acquaintance with opium first began) to 1812. And what am I doing? Taking opium. Yes, but what else? ... I have been chiefly studying German metaphysics.... And I still take opium? On Saturday nights.... And how do I find my health after all this opium-eating? In short, how do I do? Why, pretty well, I thank you, reader ...

Of course, heroin is more addictive than opium, which De Quincey took in the form of laudanum, a tincture of opium in alcohol, but the fundamental phenomena of addiction with all opiates are very similar. On his own account, De Quincey took opium for years, some four hundred times, without becoming addicted. And we also know that surgical patients, who are given opiates repeatedly for several days after operations, may acquire tolerance to them (that is to say, they require larger and larger doses to produce the same effect), and may also experience withdrawal effects if the opiates are suddenly stopped, but they do not become addicted in the sense of compulsively seeking the drug thereafter. They simply stop taking it because they no longer wish to continue.

The second of the four-volume *Encyclopedia of Drugs and Alcohol,* a reference work that can hardly be accused of skepticism towards the standard view, says this of the development of what it calls dependence:

> Susceptible persons rarely become compulsive daily users [of heroin] immediately after first use.... Susceptible persons increase the

frequency of use until it reaches once or several times daily. From first use to daily use typically takes about one year, but it may take much longer....

In the progression from initial use to daily use, heroin users learn how to inject intravenously, how to acquire the drug and injection equipment, and with some exceptions, how to conduct illegal moneymaking activities to pay for the heroin.

This is borne out by William Burroughs' first book, the auto-biographical *Junkie* (first published pseudonymously in 1953 under the title *Junk*). This book is a mixture of self-serving lies and exhibitionist frankness typical of the genre of opiate confessional. In one of his rare moments of truthfulness, probably accidental and certainly without realization of the moral significance of what he is saying, the psychopathic Burroughs writes:

> You don't wake up one morning and decide to be a drug addict. It takes at least three months' shooting twice a day to get any habit at all.

In other words, the establishment of an addiction requires a certain discipline or determination. It is not something that creeps up on you unnoticed or unannounced or all unawares. As a moment's reflection would suggest to anyone not blinded by self-interest, this fact has important and profound implications for the very concept of treatment, which in effect is metaphorical at best, a masque, veneer, pretense, or charade rather than the thing itself. For it requires as much effort to sustain an addiction, especially to opiates, as to acquire it in the first place.

The programme outlined in the *Encyclopedia* is a rigorous and demanding one, not to be undertaken lightly. It can hardly be completed, either, without considerable conscious thought on the part of the addict-to-be. It cannot just happen, like a meteorite falling on one's head. When such an addict later says that he first tried the drug under social pressure or out of mere curiosity, but before he knew where he was he was helplessly hooked, his self-exoneration is therefore not wholly to be believed. Moreover, as the *Encyclopedia* makes very clear, addiction is not synonymous with, and neither requires nor is defined by, the development of physical tolerance to the drug and the presence of withdrawal symptoms on its cessation (if it did, surgical patients would behave just like inner-city addicts).

The fundamental or defining phenomenon of addiction is said by the *Encyclopedia* to be craving, a persistent and overwhelming desire to take the drug, a desire that is obsessional and stronger than any other desire that enters or could enter the mind.

If this is so, then the explanation of addiction lies in the realm of psychology rather than of medicine, except insofar as the phenomena of psychology are ultimately reducible to those of physiology. Moreover, craving is both what is to be explained and its own explanation. We know a man craves a drug by his constant searching for it, to the exclusion of almost all other activities, and we know that he behaves in this fashion because he craves the drug.

That heroin does not "hook" the patient as a gaff hooks a boat or a lasso entangles a calf, as if the addict-to-be were but a moveable object and heroin an irresistible force, is also proved by the fact that many people who take heroin take it intermittently, much as people consume any other commodity, as and when they like. The Saturday-night indulgence of De Quincey is by no means uncommon, even when it comes to heroin. The facts that people have been found who take heroin at very infrequent intervals, as a self-awarded "treat," and that most addicts commence their addiction career by taking the drug intermittently for some considerable time before they take it three or four times a day without fail, suggest that it is truer to say that the addict hooks heroin than that heroin hooks the addict. The active principle in the exchange is the person, not the drug, and addiction is a freely chosen state: an obvious fact that is ignored by the addiction bureaucracy.

The *Encyclopedia* states that heroin addicts, at least those who emerge from the unmoneyed classes, have to learn how to raise money illegally for their heroin. At best, as we shall see, this is a half-, or rather a quarter-truth. And the reason they have to do so is because they cannot possibly be expected to stop taking heroin, mainly because if they do so, they suffer the most horrific withdrawal effects of the kind than no person could reasonably be expected to submit to voluntarily, at least unless under close medical supervision. Even then, it requires heroic, Herculean moral strength to volunteer for that terrible experience.

The Alleged Horrors of Withdrawal

But are the withdrawal symptoms from heroin (and other opiates) so very terrible? In the standard view of heroin addiction, they are. But let me quote from some of the major medical textbooks of our day:

> Although opiate withdrawal is not life threatening, patients can become extremely dysphoric. (Jay H. Stein, *Internal Medicine*, 5th edition, St. Louis: C. V. Mosby, 1999, p. 2297)

"Dysphoric" means, of course, unhappy or disgruntled, though "dysphoric" sounds very much more precise, technical, and medical: in other words, they are unhappy or disgruntled because they are not getting what they want. But, to adapt P. G. Wodehouse slightly, which of us is gruntled all the time?

The textbook continues:

> Fever, seizures, hallucinations, and delirium do not occur with opioid withdrawal and, when present, suggest either polydrug withdrawal or an associated medical illness.

By implication, therefore, withdrawal from other drugs is far more serious than withdrawal from opiates. In fact, withdrawal from alcohol is much more serious: one complication, delirium tremens, is quoted as having a death rate, without proper medical management, of 10 percent. Withdrawal from barbiturates, now rarely prescribed, is likewise dangerous, with a significant death rate. On occasion, withdrawal even from benzodiazepines (drugs such as diazepam and lorazepam) can result in symptoms identical to those of delirium tremens.

Cecil's Textbook of Medicine (21st edition, edited by Lee Goldman and J. Claude Bennett; W. B. Saunders: Philadelphia, 2001), states on page 55:

> From the patient's perspective, withdrawal from heroin is a dreaded clinical condition, a mixture of emotional, behavioral, and physical signs and symptoms. Although very unpleasant, it is not life threatening.

Note that the physical signs and symptoms appear last on the list, implying they are not of the deepest medical significance. The locution "from the patient's perspective" is also not one that commonly finds itself in such textbooks, introducing a subtle and understated element of skepticism in the description. It suggests that the doctor's point of view is different.

The *Oxford Textbook of Medicine* (4th edition, edited by David A. Warrell, Timothy M. Cox, and John D. Firth, 2003), says in volume 3, page 1339:

> Although uncomfortable, opiate withdrawal is not life threatening.

A book by Carson R. Harris, *Emergency Management of Selected Drugs of Abuse,* published by the American College of Emergency Physicians in Dallas in 2000, says on page 83:

> Although heroin withdrawal is never fatal to a healthy adult, it is an extremely uncomfortable illness.

"Although uncomfortable," "Although . . .never fatal": such locutions occur again and again, as if not a description of literal truth, but a necessary or obligatory genuflection to an organized lobby, of the kind that increasingly affects—perhaps terrorises would be a better way of putting it—the medical profession on matters of marginal medical concern.

In *Substance Abuse: A Comprehensive Textbook* (3rd edition, edited by Joyce H. Lowinson, Pedro Ruiz, Robert B. Millman and John G. Langrod; Williams and Wilkins: Baltimore, 1997), we read on page 416:

> The acute opioid withdrawal syndrome is a time-limited phenomenon, generally of brief duration. Following the abrupt termination of short-acting opioids such as heroin, morphine, or hydromorphone, withdrawal signs and symptoms usually subside on the second or third opioid-free day. Although uncomfortable for the addict, the opioid withdrawal syndrome, in contrast to the syndrome associated with the withdrawal of other drugs such as benzodiazepines and alcohol, does not pose a medical risk to the individual.

The implication is that the experience of withdrawal, shorn of all its associations, cannot explain very much about an addict's behavior.

These skeptical views are not confined to hard-hearted Anglo-American doctors. A book written by Dutchmen, R. J. M. Niesink, R. M. A. Jaspers, L. M. W. Komet and J. M. van Ree, entitled *Drugs of Abuse and Addiction: Neurobehavioral Toxicology* (Boca Raton: CRC Press, 1999) says on page 260:

> [Withdrawal from opiates is] time-limited …and not life-threatening, thus can be easily controlled by reassurance, personal attention and general nursing care without the need for any pharmacotherapy.

The authors continue:

> In some withdrawal reactions, such as barbiturate withdrawal and in severe alcohol withdrawal syndrome …, pharmacological treatment may be necessary to avoid potentially serious complications (e.g. convulsions).

Goodman and Gilman's The Pharmacological Basis of Therapeutics (10th edition, edited by Joel G. Harman and Lee E. Limbird; New York: McGraw Hill, 2001) states on page 666:

> The opioid withdrawal syndrome is very unpleasant but not life threatening.

In a large textbook devoted to the pathology of drug addiction, that is to say, to the physical sequelae of drug-taking viewed from the pathologist's angle, death from withdrawal is the dog that did not bark. *The Pathology of Drug Abuse* by Steven B. Karch (Boca Raton: CRC Press, 2002) is a minutely all-inclusive text, as perhaps the following quotation demonstrates:

> In the late 1800s, when opium smoking was still popular, the presence of cauliflower ears … was considered almost pathognomonic [diagnostic] for opium use. They were the result of lying for long periods on opium beds with hard wooden pillows.

It is unlikely that a text that includes a detail such as this would omit death from withdrawal, if it existed, for it includes death from almost every other conceivable cause. No such death is mentioned.

Likewise, *The Forensic Pharmacology of Drugs of Abuse*, by Olaf H. Drummer and Morris Odell (London: Edward Arnold, 2001) makes no mention of death from withdrawal.

Well, exactly how bad is an illness that "can be easily controlled by reassurance, personal attention and general nursing care"? An illness, moreover, whose major symptoms last but a few days, and which is likened (at its very worst) to the symptoms of flu? In the popular conception, it is dreadful beyond all description. For example, here is what the British liberal newspaper *The Observer* said of a gaol in which withdrawing addicts were given only symptomatic treatments:

> newcomers had to go "cold turkey," given only pain-killers to ease the cramps, insomnia, vomiting, shaking and sweating of withdrawal—a system compared to giving aspirin to an amputee.

"Coming straight off heroin is too hard," said the newspaper, quoting an addict-prisoner without a hint of that skepticism that it routinely applies to authorities, to a distinguished judge or scientist, for example. "You just want to die." Yes, withdrawal from opiates is more than human flesh can bear.

As it happens, I have seen a large number of withdrawing addicts in the prison in which I work. Of the several hundreds I have seen in the last decade, not a single one has ever caused me as a doctor to feel anxiety for his safety on account of his withdrawal (they sometimes have had dangerous illnesses as a result of their injecting habits, and they are often severely malnourished, starving even, but that is another matter). None has ever had a symptom requiring hospitalization, and all the genuine symptoms, never severe, have been relieved by simple, non-opiate medication.

It is true that the majority of them portray themselves to me as being in the grip of terrible suffering—suffering that they say is physical in nature, not mental. They hunch themselves up, they writhe in histrionic agony. They claim that they have experienced nothing as bad in the whole of their lives, that it is quite unendurable, and they make all kinds of threats if I do not prescribe something (by which they mean an opiate) to alleviate their suffering, threats that range from damaging or setting fire to their cells, to killing themselves, others or even me. (Alcoholics, incidentally, many of whom are in real and genuine danger, never make such threats.) And they add that when they do these things, the blame will not be theirs, but mine, because if I had done as they demanded, and prescribed what they wanted, they would never have acted in the threatened way. In fact, they very rarely do act in the threatened way. Those who say they are suicidal withdraw their threat, and tell me they were merely trying to get me to prescribe, when I suggest that they be put in what is known as an anti-ligature cell, that is to say, a cell so bare that there is nowhere from which to suspend a noose. This cell is bare also of the usual amenities, such as a kettle and a television, and the prospect of a night in it produces a confession that they were only "blagging," that is to say, trying to pull the wool over my eyes. My counter-threat, to put them in this cell, produces in most (not quite all) cases the most miraculous improvement in their mood and demeanor, and some leave my room laughing. It's all a game of poker, and they have lost, at least until they meet someone who takes everything they say at face value.

Simple observation demonstrates that much of what they say about themselves is simply not true. When, unbeknown to them, I have observed them before they entered my consulting room, and again after they have left it, they display a completely different kind of behavior to that which they exhibit once inside it. Gone is the hunched posture, the woebegone expression of martyrdom, the affecting scene of someone in extremis, or nearly so: they are talking or joking animatedly among themselves, and walk with quite a different step.

News of what the doctor is prescribing, or not prescribing, spreads at computer-like speeds among them. An addict who leaves my room, angrily expostulating about my failure to prescribe, adopting the manner of a man ready to fight the world whereas only moments before he had been near to death, claiming that I am not a doctor but a wanton murderer, likewise produces the most miraculous improvement in the bodily posture of all the addicts who enter my room soon afterwards, having heard his angry protests. They realize that the game is up, that there is no point in trying to fool me into prescribing what they want but do not really need, and therefore they abandon all pretence to be at death's door, and moderate their description of their symptoms accordingly, to something more believable. Incidentally, withdrawing alcoholics, who really are at risk of serious and dangerous withdrawal symptoms, either do not mention their distress at all, or, if they do, exaggerate it far less: in general, their self-reports correlate far better with what the doctor observes than the self-reports of opiate addicts. By the time alcoholics are really in danger, they are in no condition to complain of anything.

Not quite all the addicts whom I see exaggerate in this fashion, of course. Some, when I refuse them the medication that they request, and after I have duly explained the reasons for my refusal, smile and admit with a laugh that anyone who says that cold turkey is a terrible ordeal is lying and more than likely trying to bluff his way to a prescription. (Cold turkey is so called because of the piloerection—the gooseflesh—that is a sign of withdrawal from opiates, and "I'm turkeying," is a common way for addicts to describe their condition. In England, they also say, mixing their avian metaphors, that they're clucking, or "doing my cluck." Strictly speaking, they should be gobbling, or doing their gobble. They also say, in reference to the shivering that they sometimes experience when withdrawing, that they're rattling, or "doing my rattle." The ironical argot of the addicts is one of the few even minimally attractive aspects of their way of life.)

Although many doctors know about and have personally observed the difference in the way addicts present themselves to medical staff and the way they present themselves to each other, the significance of this difference somehow fails to affect their attitude or practice. They are like the doctors in pain clinics, who observe their patients with allegedly severe back pain running up stairs or along corridors, but draw no conclusions from it, and evince no skepticism about the stories that such patients tell. They continue to treat the distress of withdrawing addicts as if it were straightforwardly the result of physical illness. Only in this fashion can they avoid overt conflict with the patients: conflict that is both time-consuming and emotionally exhausting.

Nor is the variable way in which addicts present themselves, according to their audience, a matter of chance or adventitious observation only. It has been demonstrated experimentally. If drug addicts are interviewed by people presenting themselves as "straight," that is to say as people who do not themselves take drugs, the addicts report heavier drug use, higher expenditure on drugs, greater difficulty abstaining from drugs, and in particular worse withdrawal symptoms than if they are interviewed using the same questions by people who present themselves, by their dress, speech, and manner, as being themselves involved in drug abuse. It is not very difficult to imagine a reason for this difference, or to which kind of interviewer the addict in desire of a dose is more likely to express the literal truth of his situation. He has no motive to exaggerate the severity of his withdrawal symptoms among his peers; he has every motive to do so when he speaks to someone who, he thinks (probably rightly, alas), might be fooled into prescribing for him.

That withdrawal from opiates is not a serious medical condition is a truth universally acknowledged by doctors; but it is also a truth universally ignored, or whose significance is not much reflected upon, for reasons that I shall go into later. The large, indeed predominant, psychological component of the withdrawal syndrome is likewise well-known, but also ignored, at least in the standard view. Even in rats that have been made physically dependent upon opiates (that is to say, rats who have been administered opiates and have developed increased tolerance to the drugs and exhibit withdrawal signs when they are withheld from them), the physical signs of withdrawal are highly dependent upon the context in which it takes place. If they are removed to a new environment, different from the one in which they were first made dependent, they have far fewer signs of withdrawal than if withdrawn in the environment in which they were made dependent. This is no doubt because a new environment stimulates their curiosity, while the old environment leads them, in this case falsely, to expect further doses of opiates. And this no doubt helps to explain why it is that opiate addicts admitted to the hospital ward in which I work experience so few withdrawal symptoms that they are themselves surprised, and usually say after a couple of

days, "Is that all there is to it?" They are told from the very out-
set that we will prescribe no drugs for them unless we think it
necessary, and that we will be guided entirely by objective physical signs, that is to say, by what we see and measure, and not by
what they say regarding their symptoms, of which we will take
no notice whatever in our prescribing decisions because we know
from experience of others like them that they will exaggerate.
Moreover, we tell them, they will be allowed no visitors, because
we know that their visitors would be likely to slip them something, and they will not be permitted to leave the ward even for
an instant. In these circumstances, in which there is no possibility of their obtaining heroin or any substitute for heroin, the
patients experience no symptoms at all, or symptoms that are so
slight so as to be trivial and hardly worth mentioning. It is only
when they think that if they exhibit enough distress, or the kind
of behavior that they think that people exhibit when distressed,
that they will get what they want, that they do in fact either experience distress or exhibit such behavior (in these circumstances,
it is impossible to distinguish the two). As John Booth Davies
puts it in his *The Myth of Addiction,* "many of us will have seen
spoiled children who can writhe about the floor and make themselves sick if mummy refuses to give them another Easter egg."
Or, to quote Violet Elizabeth, a character in a famous English
series of children's stories about a naughty boy called William,
"I'll thrcream and thrcream and thrcream till I'm thick." To which
she adds the ominous rider, "I can."

The emotional and behavioral signs of which *Cecil's Textbook of Medicine* speaks therefore consist largely of the thespian
or histrionic exaggerations of the withdrawing addict, by which
he seeks to inveigle, or blackmail, or tire the doctor into prescribing what is not necessary but what he nevertheless desires. The
myth of the horrors of withdrawal serves other purposes as well,
which I shall describe later.

The Psychological Aspect of Withdrawal

The large psychological component of withdrawal from opiates
has been known for a long time and has repeatedly been shown
by experiment, as well as ignored. In the 1930s, for example,

experiments were performed to show that intravenous saline (salt solution) could be substituted for the addicts' habitual morphine without the addicts' knowledge, and they could be deceived out of their withdrawal symptoms. For example, Alfred R. Linde-smith, in his book *Addiction and Opiates,* writes:

> it has been conclusively established that under appropriate cir-cumstances addicts can be deceived into believing that they are receiving drugs and are under their influence when in fact they are not. They may also be led to believe that they are not under the influence of drugs when in fact they are.

Lindesmith then goes on to quote an experiment performed in 1930 by Dr. Charles Schultz, in which addicts were told that they would receive a reduction in their dosage of injected morphine over a seven-or fourteen-day period. The patients did not know to which group they had been assigned; and after the seventh day, some of those who were on the fourteen-day schedule but thought they were (or might have been) on the seven-day schedule, and were thus still receiving half their original dose, began to show great nervousness and restlessness, two of the most unpleasant symptoms of withdrawal. These symptoms disappeared immedi-ately when they were told that they were, in fact, still receiving morphine.

In similar fashion, two Indian doctors gave disguised opium to opium addicts who did not know that they were receiving it. They complained of pain and demanded relief, despite the fact that there were receiving their accustomed dose.

Lindesmith recounts his experience with an addict who "reported to me that he had been ... deceived in a hospital, and that when he discovered it he left at once, resenting 'their mak-ing a fool of me.' He had been getting sterile [i.e. non-opiate] hypodermics for days and was feeling quite well until an atten-dant, whom he had bribed to find out how much morphine he was getting, disclosed the truth. Instances of this kind are quite common."

Common they may be, but no one takes any notice of them or reflects for long upon their meaning. This continued, and in my view wilful, blindness to very important facts is exemplified further by a paper from the University Psychiatric Clinic of Vienna, published in 1991. The authors set out to correlate subjective reports of distress during withdrawal and objective physical signs. Oddly enough, though unsurprisingly to me, they didn't find any such correlation. There was none whatsoever. In their discussion of their findings, the authors do not even consider the question of the truthfulness of self-reports, or the importance of the social context in which such distress is reported. For them, subjective distress is objective, in the sense that it can be measured by questionnaires on analogue scales, in the same straightforward way that blood pressure or serum potassium can be measured. No problems arise in their minds about their procedure, or the layers of meaning that attach to it. And they suggest in their conclusions that doctors should henceforth take more notice of subjective reports of distress (i.e. prescribe yet more drugs), as if it were impossible that to do so would actually be to increase the motive for such reports, and even to increase the distress itself.

There is another, even more telling omission in their paper. They withdrew opiate addicts using a method known as "ultra-short opiate detoxification." This means the administration of an opiate antagonist, naloxone, under general anaesthesia, followed by continued administration of naloxone for a further forty-eight hours. This is interesting in itself, insofar as it turns a trivial medical condition, namely "natural" withdrawal from opiates, into a potentially fatal one, since quite a number of deaths are known to have occurred as a result of it, some clinics that use it having recorded as many as ten deaths. Thus zealous medicalization and the search for a technical solution to a problem that is technical only to a very minor extent has already killed a number of people.

The authors of the paper used two scales, one to measure objective signs of withdrawal, and another to measure subjective distress. As I have mentioned, there was no correlation between the two scores, but what was most interesting, though completely unnoticed by the authors, was the high level of withdrawal distress experienced by the addicts before they had even been withdrawn. Their maximum distress on the linear scale was 57, which they experienced twenty-four hours after the anaesthesia and the first dose of naloxone. However, at twenty-four hours before the anesthesia, and while they were still receiving their full dose of opiates, their score was 35, that is to say, 61 percent of the maximum score. If, as seems very likely, their distress increased in linear fashion as the time for the procedure approached (for after all, anxiety rather than true withdrawal must have been the explanation of their high score of withdrawal fully twenty-four hours before they were withdrawn, and they had been told in advance when the ultrashort withdrawal would take place), their score at time zero would have been 47, that is to say 82.5 percent of the maximum score. Even if the 10 extra points of distress they reported after the ultrashort opiate detoxification were caused wholly and solely by withdrawal as a physiological phenomenon, which seems to me unlikely since all the patients had given their informed consent to the procedure and knew exactly what was being done to them, this means that only 17.5 percent of the distress reported by the withdrawing addicts could have been due to withdrawal itself rather than to fear of withdrawal.

Interestingly, the data in the paper are presented graphically in such a fashion that the unwary might not notice that, fully twenty-four hours before any true withdrawal could have taken place, because the patients were still taking their opiates, they suffered 61 percent of the level of distress they were ever going to reach. The steep climb on the graph to the maximum level was, if not untrue exactly, misleading. This way of presenting data graphically is, or was, common in the sales propaganda of drug companies. It is not science, it is advertising.

I shall return to the question of why the authors did not notice this. Taken in conjunction with previous observations, however, it means that distress from withdrawal from opiates is overwhelmingly a social or psychological condition and not caused by observable physiological changes. And this itself has extremely important implications for practice. Assuming for a moment what cannot be altogether assumed, namely that the distress reported by withdrawing addicts is genuinely experienced and not faked or exaggerated for ulterior motives, it means that anyone who suggests that withdrawal is a serious condition, worthy of and necessitating medical attention and treatment, other than treatment of the most trivial kind, is, wittingly or not, increasing the

distress that withdrawal causes. In other words, the whole apparatus of care, doctors, nurses, psychologists, social workers, counsellors, serves not to alleviate suffering but to create and exacerbate
it. The great glory of this, from the point of view of Keynesian
economics, is that where suffering exists it is necessary to employ
doctors, nurses, psychologists, social workers, counsellors to
relieve it. (I cannot resist quoting a law first enunciated by Dr.
Colin Brewer about modern society: suffering increases to meet
the means available for its alleviation.) And thus we see a continually spiralling merry-go-round, at least with regard to withdrawal symptoms, for the alleviation of which more and more
elaborate procedures are proposed. One wouldn't have to be a
Marxist to suspect that economic interests, albeit not very powerful ones when compared with, say, the oil industry, are involved
here.

In the above sketch, I am viewing things charitably, in the
best possible light, by assuming that the reports of withdrawal
distress are not consciously dissimulated in the slightest. The
briefest acquaintance with drug addicts as a class makes this inter-
pretation unlikely, to say the least, at least in most cases.

This is not to say that withdrawal from opiates has no physiological basis whatever: clearly it has. It can be demonstrated in
laboratory animals, for example. Furthermore, properly controlled trials have demonstrated that the prescription of drugs
such as methadone can and does decrease the symptoms experienced by withdrawing drug addicts. But while these trials are double blind from the point of view of both the investigator and the
subject not knowing what the latter is receiving, they are not blind
in the sense that the subject does not know he is being withdrawn
from his original opiates, and they are therefore inferior to the
experiments performed in the 1930s. The latest science is not necessarily the best science, at least in this field. The overall understanding of the situation of the addict in modern trials is already
conditioned by his previously existing and largely false expectations. If it were not for those false expectations, the distress to be
relieved would be slight—and a trivial reduction of trivial symptoms is not in itself a great medical triumph, even less so when it
is bought at the cost, as it sometimes is, of real danger.

A major plank of the standard view is thus revealed to be very weak, indeed rotten through and through, and can bear no weight at all. Not only is this so, but it is obviously so. Yet there is little doubt that to the horrors of withdrawal are ascribed all manner of terrible consequences, not least the criminality usually associated with heroin addiction. And if there is one thing that "treatment" of addicts is supposed to do, it is to reduce their criminal propensities.

The Relation Between Heroin Addiction and Criminality

The crime associated with heroin addiction is believed on the standard view to arise from two factors. The first is the need to obtain heroin to avoid withdrawal symptoms. As we have seen, withdrawal is a trivial condition, and insofar as it is feared it is because it has been inflated in the imagination to something that intrinsically it is clearly not. Over and over again, medical writers liken withdrawal, at worst, to a dose of flu.

Actually, to compare withdrawal from opiates with influenza is absurd. Influenza is far more serious, indeed infinitely so. A large proportion of the excess number of deaths in Great Britain during the winter months is attributable to epidemics of influenza, that sometimes kill 4,000 people in that country alone (of the epidemic after the First World War, which killed up to 50,000,000 people, that is to say far more than the war itself, I shall not speak; and the current anxiety over the appearance of mutant avian flu bears me out). But we all know what flu is meant to mean in this context: an aspirin and a day or two in bed with a hot water bottle before full recovery takes place spontaneously. We ascribe no curative properties either to the aspirin or to the hot water bottle.

Let me ask the reader this: if you were given a choice between suffering a bout of flu in the above sense, or avoiding it by robbing someone in the street or breaking into a house and stealing its contents, which would you choose? The former, I hope and trust. Thus, avoidance of withdrawal does not constitute a plausible motive for the commission of crime in someone disinclined to commit crime, except to the extent that the addict believes that withdrawal is something so horrible than no one could be expected to endure it merely for the sake of a moral principle: a belief that is fostered by the very professionals whom I have blamed for increasing the suffering from withdrawal in the first place. The apparatus of care is thus the handmaiden of crime.

But, it will be argued, the addict, impelled by his craving and his necessity (however caused) to obtain his heroin, must raise the money for it somehow. A locus classicus of this kind of thinking is an article that appeared recently in the liberal British newspaper *The Guardian* by Polly Toynbee, advocating that drugs should be given to addicts free of charge so that they did not "have to" mug and burgle to obtain them, refraining from either drugs or crime not being a realistic possibility for them. The forbiddance of heroin drives up the price, and the very nature of the drug prevents the addict from pursuing gainful legal employment. Crime results as naturally as wind shakes autumn leaves from trees.

Is this really so? As usual, the standard view simplifies matters, to put it mildly. It has been known for a very long time that opiate addiction is not completely incompatible with gainful employment. In 1928, Lawrence Kolb, then the doyen of American experts on addiction, wrote of 119 of those rare addicts who had become addicts after medical prescription, of whom only twenty-nine had poor subsequent employment records:

> Judged by the output of labor and their own statements, none of the normal persons had their efficiency reduced by opium. Twenty-two of them worked regularly while taking opium for twenty-five years or more; one of them, a woman aged 81 and still alert mentally, had taken 3 grains of morphine daily for 65 years. She gave birth to and raised 6 children, and managed her household affairs with more than average efficiency. A widow, aged 66, had taken 17 grains of morphine daily for most of 37 years. She is alert mentally but is bent with age and rheumatism. However, she does physical labor every day and makes her own living.

The heroin addict who makes his own living is likewise not unknown. While it is very difficult to believe that addiction to heroin or to anything else could make a working life easier, unless it be by well-judged and titrated tranquilizing effect, neither too little nor too much but just right, it does not make it impossible, and therefore cannot be said to compel the commission of crime.

If addiction to heroin were itself the cause of crime, on account of the high price of heroin, one might expect the amount of crime committed by individual heroin addicts to decrease as the price decreased. This is not necessarily so. The total amount of crime committed by heroin addicts both individually and collectively might increase, because it is well-known that the price of psychoactive substances, nicotine in tobacco and alcohol among them, affects the total level of their consumption in society. Thus a decrease in price might mean an addict chose to increase his consumption rather than cut down on his need to commit crime to fund his habit: but that would be a matter of choice rather than of compulsion.

Besides, the life of a drug-addicted criminal is actually quite busy, though it is rarely very successful, from the purely economic point of view. He has not only to steal, but—if he does so to raise money to buy his heroin, drug dealers not accepting payment in kind—to dispose of whatever he steals. It might very well take less effort just to go out to work, except that most employment requires punctuality and reliability. Thus he has not only to steal, but to steal continually, according to the picture painted by holders of the standard view. Even quite valuable items, such as video machines, fetch very low sums on the black market, because our society is nearly saturated with them. Thus the addict has to work quite hard not to go to work.

While it is true that heroin addicts commit many crimes, and a far greater proportion of them have criminal records than others of their age and social class, the relationship between crime and heroin addiction is more complex than the simple, standard view would suggest. For example, one investigation established that in the group of addicts studied there was no correlation between the amount of heroin an individual addict consumed and his criminal activities, as there should have been if the crime committed by addicts was simply and solely to obtain money for the drug. The best predictor of theft by addicts was found to be the variety of crimes they had already committed, which accounted for far more of the variance between them than their actual drug use.

I confirmed these findings in the prison in which I work. I asked a hundred drug-addicted prisoners, interviewed on their reception into prison on a new sentence or remand, when in their lives they had first been given a prison sentence. A little later in the interview, so that they would not realize the purpose of my question, I asked them when they had first taken heroin.

Sixty-seven of them had been to prison before they had ever tried heroin. Eight of them claimed to have taken heroin for the first time while they were in prison, usually not for the first time. In Britain, unless the first crime for which someone is convicted is a serious one, which is unusual, a man has to commit several, indeed many, crimes before he is incarcerated for the first time. Criminals are convicted for one in five to fifteen crimes that they commit, and in Britain usually have been convicted ten times before they receive a prison sentence. That is to say, many of the heroin addicts I saw in prison might have committed between fifty and several hundred crimes before they ever took heroin.

As for those who start taking heroin in prison, they can hardly claim that their subsequent criminality was caused by heroin addiction, unless they also claim what is not very plausible, that had it not been for their decision to take heroin in prison they would have gone straight.

In other words, heroin-taking is more a consequence than a cause of criminality, and the decision to take heroin, whether in prison or outside, is therefore the conscious choice of a criminal lifestyle. (Interestingly, the argot of the housing projects and other slums is increasingly the argot of prison.) A criminal mentality causes heroin addiction more than heroin addiction causes criminality. The standard view gets the causative relationship, if any, exactly the wrong way round. This is borne out by a study of the effects of prescribing methadone to intravenous drug addicts in Sheffield, England: those of them (29 percent) who took the drug regularly, as prescribed, and ceased taking heroin, reduced their levels of acquisitive crime from 13 per month to a mere 3 per month. Fine upstanding citizens who steal only 36 times per year, despite being given their drugs gratis! It seems that it is indeed lucky for heroin addicts that there is no justice in the world, for if there were, they would all be permanently in prison.

Of course, that a debased way of life such as heroin addiction should exercise an appeal or fascination, and on such a large scale, might well be a terrible indictment of our society as well as of the individuals who indulge in it. If the best option in life for young men and women seems to them to be the squalor of heroin addiction and intermittent incarceration, then it is a sad reflection on the choices that they believe are available to them, often because no one has taken the trouble to offer them anything else. They are willing to exchange a life of respectable impoverishment and the hope of gradual improvement for the repeated oblivion and forgetfulness with which heroin provides them. Many addicts admit to me that they continue to take the drug not to avoid the withdrawal effects, as the standard view suggests, but continually "to forget." I shall later describe what it is that, all too understandably, they do not wish to recall.

The Alleged Need for Treatment

The final plank of the standard view is the need for treatment. Addicts cannot possibly escape their chains without professional assistance. This is a view as eagerly adopted by the addicts themselves as by those who set out, ostensibly, to help them. So large is the number of addicts, however, that it has quite swamped or overwhelmed the services set up to help them, even as those services expand continually. Addicts often have to wait an age (and anything longer than a few hours or a day is an age to an addict) before they can be taken on by a clinic. They have, in their own view, no option but to continue to take heroin.

On this view, of course, heroin addiction is a bona fide illness, and it makes as little sense to expect an addict to cure himself by taking thought as it would be to demand of a patient with tuberculosis to stop coughing up blood by deciding not to do so any more. Addiction is thus something that happens to you, not something that you do. Hence the need for expert assistance arises, and it is as cruel to make addicts wait for medical assistance as it would be to make consumptives wait for it.

But is this really true? Once again, we find that it is not. There is a famous historical example, from the not very distant past, that demonstrates that it is not true. During the Vietnam War, thousands of American soldiers, especially towards the end, addicted themselves to heroin. It is not very difficult to imagine why American soldiers found heroin attractive: their life was, like that of most soldiers during a war, 99 percent boredom and 1 percent terror. The supply found its market soon enough. (It was even said that the Vietnamese communists spread addiction deliberately to weaken the resolve and capacity of American soldiers.)

The Encyclopedia of Drugs and Alcohol (Volume 3, pages 1244 to 1245) described what happened. Forty-three percent of American servicemen had tried heroin, and 20 percent of them qualified as addicts. What happened to them when they went home? Only one in eight of the addicts continued with his addiction after return to the United States, and by two and three years after their return, the addiction rates among those who had served were no higher than among those who qualified for the draft but did not serve in Vietnam.

And what help or services did these thousands of addicts receive when they returned home? For all intents and purposes, it varied between very little and none. They simply stopped taking heroin and did not resume.

You might think that this historical experience was of cardinal importance for those who consider the problem of drug addiction. It cannot be said that it is an obscure or unknown fact. Here is what another well-known text, *Handbook of Substance Misuse: Neurobehavioral Pharmacology* (edited by Robert E. Tarter, Robert T. Ammerman and Peggy J. Ott; New York: Plenum, 1998) says about it, strictly en passant, on page 370. The author is arguing that withdrawal of the drug alone is not enough, that more elaborate procedures and treatment are necessary to stop addicts from taking their drugs:

> In general, the "detoxification only" approach is not appropriate; it is followed by relapse in most cases.... However, notable exceptions have been reported from Vietnam War veterans, addicts treated in corrections systems [by which the author means not treated], and those who adopt a new religion and lifestyle.

And that is all—the rest is silence. There is no reflection on the meaning of an illness that can be cured in so unorthodox a fashion: return home from serving as a soldier abroad, incarceration, or religious conversion. Try that on cancer. These are not miracles, incidentally: they are commonplaces. The latest religion or faith to effect a cure of addiction is the now outlawed Falun Gong movement in China—opiate addiction having re-emerged in China with the greater freedom of people to do as they wish.

I hesitate now to mention another historical example, in case I should be taken to be advocating the methods used: namely Mao's China after he took power. In 1949, China had more opiate addicts than the rest of the world put together, the exact figure being in the nature of things unknowable, but possibly in the region of 20,000,000.

In short order, Mao gave addicts a strong motive to give up and the rest of the population a strong motive not to start. He shot the dealers out of hand, and any such addicts who did not give up their habit. The carrot for addicts was life and the stick was death. It would not be going too far to say that, within a mere three years, Mao produced more cures than all the drug clinics in the world before or since, or indeed to come. He was the greatest drug worker in history.

The point of this story is not to advocate a repetition of Mao's methods on our soil, but to demonstrate that, when a motive is sufficiently strong, not merely some, but many, indeed millions, of addicted people can abandon their addiction, without the whole paraphernalia of the help that is necessary on the standard view of the problem, and that the drug addict refers to when he says that he would give up, if he had "the help."

Not only does the example from Mao's China accord with the rather less draconian example of the American servicemen returning from Vietnam, it accords with the simple fact that many heroin addicts do abandon their habit spontaneously—by no means all of them continue forever, or die from the consequences of it. An item in a recent edition of *The Lancet* written by a family doctor makes this point:

> When a patient came into the surgery recently about some mundane problem, I recalled that the last time I had seen him several years ago—he had told me about his long-standing heroin habit. He was now looking conspicuously healthy and well groomed and he confirmed that he had given it up. So what happened? He said he had "just got fed up with it." How had he done it—methadone,

rehab, religion? No, he just decided one day that he had "had enough" and stopped. Just like that? Pretty much—he was "a bit rough" for a few days, but then "that was it."

The author goes on to say:

> I have met more people who have succeeded in giving up drugs through their own efforts than I have those who have emerged successfully from treatment programmes.

Now of course this is not evidence in the statistical sense—it is one man's experience merely; and not only is his sample unlikely to be representative of addicts as a whole, but his recall of his own sample may be faulty. Nevertheless, the story of his reformed addict is instructive, when taken in conjunction with the historical examples. Historical example, therefore, and individual experience, render trivial, redundant, and futile the elaborate researches of hundreds, if not of thousands, of scientists, doctors and sociologists, be they ever so ingenious and interesting in themselves. People can give up taking opiates if they wish to do so, and they wish to do so if they have a sufficient reason for doing so, be it positive or negative.

It might be argued in the case of Maoist China that the motive provided was very extreme, and so it was. But it acted through the imagination, and thereby upon behavior, nonetheless. Let us suppose that Mao, on coming to power, had decided to eliminate appendicitis by the same means: would it have made sense? Such means might possibly have inhibited people from complaining of the symptoms of appendicitis, or seeking medical assistance when they suspected they had appendicitis, but they would not have eliminated the condition itself. To treat an addiction as if it were a medical illness pure and simple, susceptible of medical cure, is absurd: and yet that is what the concept of "help" implies, that there is some procedure that can be carried out that will "cure" the patient, even if the supposed cure involves a lot of talking. I shall return to the absurd pas de deux between the addict and his "therapist" in due course.

Actually, as I have already indicated, some of the addicts whom I see in the prison recognize that they need a motive to give up their habit. They have no choice but to give up now, they say, because a baby is either on the way or has just been born to them.

This is an implicit recognition of the fact that a motive is both a necessary and sufficient condition for them to give up. In this particular instance, the fact that their girlfriend is about to have, or has just had, a baby, often not the first, does not, in the event, provide such a motive. The reason for this is that the addicts are drawn from a stratum of British society in which eventual, and often swift, abandonment of children by their fathers is now not merely common but almost universal. The idea that a father has an inescapable responsibility of any kind to his offspring is now so alien that not even the mothers of their children believe it. A baby in this stratum is not an expression of love between two people, or even the fulfilment of a social obligation, but an instrument of power or a supposed means of answering an existential problem, such as boredom, lovelessness, and meaninglessness. Where even the non-addicted fathers abandon their children, it is not to be expected that the addicted will behave better or more responsibly. Babies are exciting and important for a time, but not for long. The motive does not last long, and rarely survives the first demand for financial maintenance.

The point about the social (or anti-social) world in which so many of my addicts live is that it provides almost no motives for them to give up. Even the avoidance of death is not a motive for them because, while most of them know of people who have died as a result of the habit, they also believe in the almost infinite, and certainly very great, power of medicine to save life. If they know people who have died, they also know people who have been saved, for example after an overdose of heroin. The risk-taking nature of young people is well-known and observable on our roads. The avoidance of a small absolute chance of death is not sufficient to deter them, although the relative risk of death compared with that of non-addicts may be extremely high.

Even if treatment, using the word in its metaphorical sense, is not necessary, it is frequently given. And the most frequent form of treatment is the substitution of one drug for another. If you can't beat it, alter it.

The Nature of Treatment

The object of treatment, so called, is either the abstention of the addicted person, or if that proves to be "impossible" (again I use the word metaphorically), harm reduction. This means that if a person insists upon taking heroin by intravenous injection, you provide him with the needles and syringes so that he should not suffer the transmissible diseases from needles and syringes used by other addicts. (In Canadian prison recently, the authorities have offered to provide prisoners with tattoos to prevent them from tattooing themselves, a procedure that involves risk. They must, however, choose non-racist, non-violent designs.) This policy certainly seems to reduce the chances of an addict contracting HIV or Hepatitis B and C. If a person persists in taking opiates, and in committing crime to obtain the money to pay for them, you provide him with free opiates so that he commits no more crime. And so on and so forth, always in the direction of accommodation of the habit, of course.

The addict is not to be confronted directly with the consequences of his own actions; in modern society, we want our risk and our safety too. It is the modern equivalent of eating one's cake and having it.

The benefits of what is called risk-reduction are tangible, or at least measurable. The benefits of refusing to reduce risk are intangible or philosophical, though it is possible in the long run that they would translate into tangible, or measurable, ones. When self-indulgent actions, such as taking heroin, are deprived of some of their worst consequences, it is hardly to be wondered at that they spread like wildfire through a population. If consequences are removed from enough actions, then the very concept of human agency evaporates, life itself becomes meaningless, and is thenceforth a vacuum in which people oscillate between boredom and oblivion. They have nothing to hope for and nothing to fear; they are more likely to seek the intermittent oblivion of opiate addiction.

Harm reduction as a policy is inherently infantilizing of the population: it assumes that the authorities are, and ought to be, responsible, for the ill-consequences of what people insist upon doing. A recent case in a Canadian women's prison illustrates this. A prisoner, addicted to opiates, was given a dose of methadone to prevent her from suffering; but so slight was the suffering that she anticipated, no doubt from her previous experience, from withdrawal from opiates—the suffering that supposedly justified the prescription in the first place—that she voluntarily vomited up her methadone, to give it, or more likely to sell it, to another prisoner who was not an addict. The latter drank the former's vomit, and died as a consequence.

Who was to blame? The prison authorities, of course. The relatives of the deceased immediately sued them. There is thus no reasonable expectation that people should not drink one another's vomitus, or that, if they do, they should take the consequences themselves. We are all children, and the authorities are our parents.

This is utilitarianism made policy. It infantilizes the subject, however, and treats him as if he were not responsible for his own actions. In fact, experience shows that the subject is not quite such an automaton as is often made out (a subject to which I shall return): for example, in the prison in which I work, the vast majority of heroin addicts who inject themselves with the drug give up injecting because clean needles are not made available to them, and they are aware of the dangers of injecting with needles that others have already used. This suggests that, at the very least, prisoners are conscious, and indeed self-conscious, beings. Of course, a small number of such addicts continue to inject, putting themselves at risk, and it is this small minority upon whom policy-makers, always biased in favour of more official intervention, focus their attention. There is nothing an official hates more than a person who makes up his own mind.

My experience is not unique. It has been found in formal surveys in Scotland, for example, that the majority of injecting addicts do not inject once they are in prison. They know what they are doing. Nevertheless, it is up to the authorities to prevent prisoners from starting to take drugs in prison. A paper in the *British Medical Journal* stated that "Prisons need to understand how initiation [into injecting] occurs and to support non-injectors ...so that they can avoid starting to inject inside." The very language of this paper turns those who choose to inject heroin in prison for the first time into billiard balls impacted upon by other billiard balls.

The *ne plus ultra* of the harm-reduction philosophy, however, is to be found in the policy of retoxification introduced in some Scottish prisons. Addicts who stop taking heroin in prison sometimes celebrate their release—within hours, not days—by taking an injection of heroin. As they have lost their physiological tolerance to the drug in the meantime, and as they often take the dose to which they were accustomed before they were sent to prison, quite a number of them die. Others end up in intensive care units of local hospitals, where their lives are saved.

It is not always or even usually a lack of knowledge about the facts of tolerance that leads them to this dangerous behavior. I recall a prisoner who was a heroin addict and who was due for release in the near future, whom I warned of the dangers of reduced tolerance. The day following his release, I met him again in the hospital in which I also work, and which is next door to the prison; he had taken heroin and had briefly needed artificial ventilation as a result.

"Did you remember what I told you?" I asked.

"Yes."

"Didn't you believe me?"

"Yes, I believed you."

"Then why did you take no notice?"

"I met up with my old friends."

The anticipated pleasure was great, the price was right, and the temptation strong. All of us know what it is like to give in to temptation, and to that extent the man was deserving of our compassion. It was right to save his life, but would it have been right to tell him that he had done no wrong, or that like Luther he could have done no other? Would not that have been to turn him into something less than a man?

This is what the prison retoxification scheme seeks to do. Recognizing that some prisoners like the one I have just described are inclined to die as a result of their celebratory heroin injection (indeed, their death rate in the two weeks following release from prison may be thirty-four times as high as at any other time outside prison), their tolerance to opiates is deliberately increased in prison after a period of abstinence so that they may safely inject on their release. Thus their decision to inject themselves is treated like a natural fact that is independent of human volition, which is to say that they are not like you and me, who for good or ill make up our own minds about what to do and suffer the consequences. They are mere objects, to be manipulated in a technocratic fashion, to be given drugs as a machine is oiled, so that it won't seize up; and while this is dehumanizing, and puts them in a humiliating position *vis-à-vis* their would-be benefactors, it also gives them a certain weak-minded gratification of the kind to which they have already proved themselves susceptible. A vicious circle of mutual pretence between benefactor and recipient is set up, a matter to which I shall return. Meanwhile, the fact that the overall death rate of addicts during the time they are sent to prison plus the two weeks after their release is not greater than an equivalent period outside prison altogether suggests that imprisonment without release exerts a life-preserving effect upon them. It is their release into freedom that kills them, not their imprisonment; a sad commentary upon their lives no doubt, but one whose philosophical, ethical, and practical significance entirely escapes the harm-avoidance drug treatment school of thought.

The Logic of Methadone

The idea of the most common method of treatment (it would be tedious to put this term always in quotation marks, but I hope the reader will take them as read) is substitution of heroin for a drug called methadone.

This substance, which is most often taken in syrup form, but is also available as an injection and as pills, is a synthetic opiate first developed in Germany just before the beginning of the Second World War. The most commonly accepted, though not necessarily true, version of its invention is that the Nazis, fearing that their supply of natural opiates would be cut off during hostilities, and aware that the Reichsmarschall Hermann Goering was a morphine addict liable to withdrawal symptoms if his supply of heroin was interrupted, asked the German pharmaceutical industry to develop a synthetic opiate that freed Germany from the need to import, and Goering from his fears. (One website, with the revealing address heroinhelper.com/bored/celebrities, states that "Goering is most remembered as the leader of the Luft-waffe, but he is an excellent example of how little a problem opium addiction is, when the opioid is legal and readily available.") It has often been asserted also that one of the American brand names for methadone, Dolophine, is in honor of the political leader in whose regime its discovery was made. This is strenuously denied by defenders of methadone, who claim that the drug, the patent for which passed to the allies as a spoil of war, was so called by combining two French words, *douleur,* pain, and *fin,* end, that is to say the end of pain. If so, it was a remarkably insensitive play on words, since the drug in Nazi Germany had been named in honour of Adolf Hitler, and the word is at least as likely to conjure up Adolf as *fin de douleur.* In Austria and Germany, at any rate, they have not taken the same verbal risk. In Austria, methadone is branded as Heptadone, and in Germany as Methaddict (itself a name not without interesting connotations).

Still, the historical origin of a drug, or the association of ideas stimulated by its name, is hardly relevant to its medical value. No one, after all, objected to the discovery of the first anti-bacterial sulphonamide—Prontosil—let alone sulphonamides as a class of drugs, because it was discovered in Nazi Germany. But yet the unease about the origin of methadone persists. This is how *The Encyclopedia of Drugs and Alcohol* (Vol 2, page 542), describes the history of the discovery of heroin:

> In Germany, in 1898, H. Dresser introduced ... a new drug—3,6-diacetylmorphine—into medical use; it was named there by the Bayer Company, which produced and marketed it, heroin (presumably from *heroisch,* meaning "heroical"), because it was more potent than morphine.

And here is what it says (on page 671 of the same volume) about the history of methadone:

> Methadone (Dolophine) serves an important place in the history of opioid analgesics, since it is one of the first synthesized agents (1939).

Not much historical context there.

Methadone has a long half-life: that is to say, it takes a rel-atively long time for the body to metabolize and excrete it. Thus it produces its effect over twenty-four hours or more, and is taken but once a day, whereas the effects of heroin last only a few hours, so that the addict may take it up to three or four times daily. It is said not to produce the euphoria that heroin produces, which from the point of view of treatment, though not from the addict's point of view, is also said to be an advantage. Here, of course, there is a contradiction, for it is often asserted that opiate addicts, once they have become addicted to the drug, experience no eupho-ria, but continue to take their drug only in order to feel normal, that is to say, not in a state of withdrawal. In this way, they are exculpated from the charge of irresponsible hedonism, of actu-ally enjoying their wretched habit, of robbing and burgling to pay for their pleasure. Robbing and burgling to avoid their pain seems somehow so much more meritorious, or at least less rep-rehensible, than robbing and burgling to enjoy for a few hours a fool's paradise. But in actual fact, many addicts will admit that they continue to derive pleasure from heroin, and that is precisely why they continue.

When a heroin addict is prescribed methadone, the object is to stabilize his life. Thenceforth (it is hoped), he will cease, or at least reduce, his consumption of heroin, and all the behavior necessary to obtain it. This will reduce his chances of contract-ing HIV and Hepatitis B and C. (Of course, this applies only to those who inject heroin: those who smoke it are at no greater risk of infection with these viruses than non-addicts.) Finally, his sup-ply of methadone being either free or very cheap, he will no longer feel the need to commit crime "to feed his habit," as the cant phrase has it.

Controlled trials have indeed demonstrated the advantages of methadone substitution therapy. If you divide a group of addicts into two, and give half of them methadone and the other half a placebo, then those in receipt of methadone will reduce their con-sumption of heroin and commit fewer crimes, both by compari-son with their own previous records and by comparison with those in receipt of placebo. As far as the drug addiction estab-lishment is concerned, this is QED: in essence, all you have to do to defeat heroin addiction as an individual and social problem is to distribute more and more methadone in more and more clinics to more an more addicts.

And, one might add, in higher and higher doses. Similar trials have demonstrated that big doses of methadone are more effective in preventing "relapse" (that is to say, a resumption of heroin-taking by the addicts) than smaller doses. In a way, this makes perfect physiological sense. The opiate receptors in the brain are swamped by higher, but not by smaller, doses; therefore, if a patient on a higher dose of methadone takes some heroin, he experiences no pleasure from it because it can have no effect upon his brain. His motive for taking heroin is therefore less than that of someone taking a smaller dose.

The idea of methadone substitution has become virtually an unassailable orthodoxy, the subject, for example, of a National Institute of Health consensus statement, which occupies roughly the same position in the mental economy of the medical profession as a papal bull in that of the clergy in pre-reformation Europe. But the logic of it all seems to me to be distinctly flawed, at least when it is instituted as social policy.

The success, at least partial, of treating heroin addicts with methadone, and the fact that there is a dose-response curve (that is to say, the higher the dose, the stronger the effect), suggests to the addiction establishment that heroin addiction is therefore a bona fide medical condition, what one paper in *The New England Journal of Medicine* called "a chronic, relapsing disorder," rather like gout, perhaps, or rheumatoid arthritis, the cause of whose fluctuations is as yet unknown.

Let us, then, perform a little thought experiment. Suppose we had a population of burglars, whom we divided into two (admittedly the experiment could not easily be double blind). The first group, when caught, receives $10,000,000; the second is given conventional "treatment," i.e., jail. It would not be very unlikely or difficult to establish that the first group's rate of recidivism (or relapse, to give crime a medical cast) would be very much lower than the second group's, at least until the money ran out. Of course, as with methadone treatment, the response would not be 100 percent, because there are no doubt some burglars who do it for the sheer hell, that is to say, the joy, of it. But it would also be possible to show a dose-response curve. Five hundred dollars might prevent relapse for a week; $5,000 for a month; and so on and so forth. Moreover, you could fiddle around with the treatment *ad infinitum,* giving burglars benefits in kind, for example, furniture and groceries, or fast red sports cars and a free subscription to a fuel station. Some treatments would undoubtedly work better than others; some would not work at all. Would this make burglary a disease?

Likewise, progressive amputation of digits and limbs, conducted with all the paraphernalia of modern surgery (and thus with all the appearance of a genuine medical treatment), might suppress burglary in burglars. There would, indeed, be a proper dose-response curve: the more of a burglar you amputated, the more effective amputation would be in reducing his burglary. But all the surgery in the world would not make burglary a medical condition or amputation a treatment for it.

Lest this strike the reader as too far-fetched, let me assure him or her that in fact criminal recidivism has been regarded by some criminologists as a form of addiction. I have read a paper in which repeated car theft (and in my prison I have met car thieves who claim to have stolen hundreds of vehicles) was described as an addiction, and it came complete with a demonstration of possible neural mechanisms in the brain not to prove it, such proof being impossible, but to give to it the patina of scientific respectability. Even more remarkable, given the obscurity of this theorizing, recidivist car thieves in the prison (one of whom was serving approximately four hours' incarceration for every car he claimed to have stolen) have asked me whether I thought, as they did, that they were addicted to car theft, the theorizing of the criminologists presumably having filtered down to what we would nowadays call the vehicle-stealing community, though network would be a more accurate term. By analogy, therefore, the treatment of addiction to stealing vehicles would be the provision of a vehicle: not perhaps a Porsche (the heroin of cars), but a small and reliable Japanese saloon (the methadone of cars).

The standard view of addiction's argument for the expansion of drug addiction services is that they are currently too small and restricted to treat the number of addicts in society. For example, one paper in *The Journal of the American Medical Association,* pointed out, and implicitly lamented, that the "current narcotic treatment system is able to provide the most effective medical treatment for opioid dependence to only 170,000 of the 810,000 'opioid-dependent individuals' in the United States" (a low estimate by comparison with a paper in the *New England Journal* only eleven months before, which gave a figure of 980,000 "long-term users"). The solution, for the authors of the paper, was to allow what is currently forbidden, namely for primary care physicians in the United States, and not merely designated narcotic treatment facilities, to prescribe methadone to opioid-addicted or -dependent or long-term-using persons. In other words, if only we could prescribe enough methadone to enough addicts, the problem would be solved. The addicts would beat their needles into ploughshares, and all would be right with the world. Treatment with substitution therapy is not only beneficial for the individual treated, but is good for the public health.

The analogy, I suppose, is with pulmonary tuberculosis. This disease is spread by a susceptible person breathing in the germs expelled by an infected person's cough. To treat an infected person, therefore, is both to cure him as an individual and to reduce the chances of the spread of the disease.

Is the treatment of heroin addicts with methadone, or any other substitute drug, like this? By reducing one addict's propensity to take illicit heroin and to commit crime, are you really reducing the total consumption of illicit heroin and drug-addiction associated crime in society? Does this really reflect the experience of the past three decades in most western societies?

Let us perform another little thought experiment. Suppose for a moment that you are a heroin addict and that I am your dealer. Suppose also that one day you come to me to tell me that you have attended the local drug clinic, are now in receipt of a prescription for methadone, and that henceforth you will not require my services. What do I do with the heroin I have earmarked for you? Do I flush it with a sigh down the nearest water closet, and lament my loss of profit? Or do I do my very best to find someone else to buy it, do I do a little market development? I think the answer is obvious.

In other words, what we end up with (at best) is a methadone addict as well as a heroin addict, whereas we had only a heroin addict before. Does not this picture fit what has actually happened in most western societies better than what would have happened had the treatment of tuberculosis model been correct? Does this not explain why treatment of heroin addiction is like the rock that Sisyphus had perpetually to push up the hill, until it rolled backwards once he nearly reached the summit? Neither the quadrupling of methadone prescriptions in Britain between 1982 and 1992, nor the doubling of them in America between 1999 and 2001, had any effect on the scale of the problem. Yet in all the papers about methadone (or other substitution) therapy, I have never seen this most obvious thought considered even for a moment.

While recently discussing methadone treatment with a medical true believer (I use the words advisedly) who was also a public health official, I pointed out that, in order to demonstrate a reduction in supposedly drug-related crime caused by the prescription of methadone to addicts, it is not sufficient to demonstrate a reduction in crime committed by those individuals alone. He reacted with something akin to a cry of pain: You're challenging the consensus, he said, as if to do so were automatically to be wrong, or, worse still, wicked. The apparatchik mentality is far from unique to the former Soviet Union.

The fact that methadone substitution therapy, or any such substitution therapy, might actually contribute to rather than prevent the spread of heroin addiction does introduce a genuine ethical dilemma into medical practice. The doctor is usually the agent of his individual patient rather than of society as a whole, and it is his duty to do what is best for that patient rather than what is best for society. Attempts to make doctors responsible to society rather than to their patients are generally one of the hallmarks of totalitarianism.

But the doctor cannot be Pontius Pilate either, and ought to acknowledge the consequences of his actions. Moreover, methadone and other drug substitution treatments are often justified on public health grounds, for example, in a publication of the British Advisory Council on the Misuse of Drugs, entitled

"AIDS and Drug Misuse Update Report," which says, "The benefit to be gained from oral methadone maintenance programmes both in terms of individual and public health and cost effectiveness has now been clearly demonstrated." Statements such as the following are routinely made, as if repetition were itself proof of truth: "Treatments such as methadone maintenance are costly, particularly because of duration of treatment, but they are still substantially cheaper than the cost to the community of the active or incarcerated drug misuser." Note how it is assumed, without proof, and against the reflections of common sense, that the results of clinical trials with a limited number of addicts are transferable directly to the whole of society.

It is in any case a moot point, that is still much debated, whether the prescription of methadone has caused more deaths than it has saved, for it is a very dangerous drug. A teaspoonful is enough to kill a baby; 30 millilitres (six teaspoonsful) have been enough to kill an adult who is not accustomed to taking opiates, though it usually takes a little more. Where methadone is prescribed in such a fashion that the daily dose is not consumed in front of a pharmacist or other reliable observer, considerable quantities of it are diverted on to the open market. In my city, the price of methadone is not high: about $1.80 for ten millilitres. This low price could be the consequence either of a light demand, or of a heavy supply.

It is accepted even by its proponents that methadone substitution is not a panacea, even for that minority for whom it is prescribed. In the best centers, up to a quarter of the addicts treated with methadone continue to take heroin, and in some centers it is more than a half. Since it is also known that patients with less chaotic backgrounds and less disordered personalities respond better than those with more chaotic backgrounds and more disordered personalities, some of the differences between centers may be attributed to differences in the characteristics of their patients, rather than to differences in any element of the treatment itself.

That the prescription of methadone does not altogether stop criminal acts by addicts is demonstrated by the presence in our prisons of many people who were prescribed the drug before they committed the offense and were convicted. In my experience, the majority of prisoners who were prescribed methadone before conviction were taking heroin and often crack or cocaine as well, usually unbeknown to the people prescribing methadone for them. While they are admittedly a selected sample of the addicts who are prescribed methadone, not representative of those addicts as a whole, they are not an insignificant sample. In Glasgow, for example, approximately a quarter of addicts prescribed methadone are convicted of a criminal offense annually; and given the inefficient nature of the British criminal justice system, the proportion who ought to be convicted is probably very much higher. Thus there is at the very least a substantial minority of addicts prescribed methadone for whom the treatment does no good whatsoever, either in reducing their criminality or the resort to other drugs. Even where it is clear to the prescriber that his prescription is ineffective, however, he continues it, for reasons that I shall later discuss.

The general hospital in which I worked treated about one patient a week who was prescribed methadone, which is about 5 percent of all the people prescribed methadone in the city. (There were two other similar hospitals in the city that probably treated as many such patients, making 15 percent of people prescribed methadone in all.) They were treated either for overdose of methadone or for complications arising from continued injection with heroin, such as deep vein thrombosis, pulmonary embolus, abscesses, or subacute bacterial endocarditis. In the vast majority of cases, their urine tested positive for a variety of other drugs, including cannabis, cocaine, heroin, codeine, and amphetamines. The hospital nevertheless came under increasing political pressure, exerted by true-believing doctors, to continue to prescribe methadone for these patients while they remained in hospital, despite the fact that they had taken overdoses of methadone and continued to take heroin and other illicit drugs, which was why they were in hospital in the first place, and despite the evident fact that methadone was neither preventing harm from coming to them nor stopping their use of illicit drugs. In one case, a patient arranged for a member of the staff of his drug addiction clinic to come to the hospital and surreptitiously deliver his methadone to him while he was still in hospital, medically a very dangerous thing to have done and a gross breach of medical ethics. Methadone has become more a religion than a treatment.

Substantial numbers of people are killed by methadone. The exact numbers are difficult to ascertain, and it is impossible to be dogmatic about whether more people proportionately die as a consequence of taking methadone than of taking heroin. The fact that it is impossible to be sure in either direction, however, suggests that methadone is not very effective, even if the harm-reduction philosophy is accepted.

One of the reasons it is so difficult to decide the question is that it is not always possible to decide what constitutes a death by methadone. Most people who die with methadone in their blood have also taken alcohol or, more especially, benzodiazepines, the class of tranquilizer to which diazepam (brand name Valium) belongs. This latter appears to be a lethal combination; its lethality, which has been long evident, has failed to deter doctors from prescribing it. Even if it so deter did, however, it is far from certain that methadone-associated deaths would cease or even decline by very much. There is much diversion of diazepam on to the open market, and takers of methadone are, virtually by definition, adepts at finding illicit drugs on the open market. In other words, those who prescribe methadone, and who claim to be such realists with regard to the behavior of heroin addicts, ought to accept that those to whom they prescribe methadone are likely to seek other drugs in dangerous combinations. Since their philosophy is to make themselves responsible for the actions of those who come under their purview, they cannot simply deny responsibility for deaths associated with methadone, even where they resulted from combinations of drugs some of which they did not themselves prescribe.

Whatever the finer points of the question, it is not difficult to find evidence of a considerable toll caused by methadone. In Britain as a whole, for example, where methadone is never prescribed for anything other than opiate addiction, the number increased seven fold between 1982 and 1992. In Scotland alone in 1998, there were 114 deaths in which heroin was directly implicated. There were 64 deaths in which methadone was directly implicated. Since at most a third of the number of heroin addicts receive a prescription for methadone, these figures could be taken to suggest that methadone is more dangerous than heroin, though in fact the figures do not permit this straightforward conclusion, since some of the deaths were probably caused by the diversion of methadone to people who had never been prescribed it. At the very least, however, the figures make clear that methadone is not a profoundly life-saving drug, such as penicillin was when it was first introduced. Diversion for sale of methadone, incidentally, demonstrates that the decision-making faculties of addicts, if not those of doctors, remain intact. They are able to choose their course of action.

According to the coroner for the City of Dublin, there were 255 drug-associated deaths in the years 1998—2000. Of these 157 were associated with heroin and 144 with methadone, and therefore some were associated with both taken at the same time. Again, benzodiazepines were taken in 70 percent of cases; and again, while these figures allow of no definite statement as to whether methadone kills or saves, and a true analysis would have to include the number of cases of AIDS and fatal Hepatitis B and C infections prevented by the prescription of methadone (but also caused by the possible increase in heroin addiction promoted by the prescription of methadone, something that is never done in the literature), they indicate that methadone is very far from a panacea, and it is perfectly possible that methadone is responsible for more deaths than it prevents. In Dublin, as elsewhere, only a minority of those who take, or have ever taken, heroin are prescribed methadone.

In Manchester, none of the deaths by overdose in 1985 was associated with methadone. By 1994, 30.6 percent of them were. (Interestingly, the same paper in the *British Medical Journal* shows that, despite a fifteen-fold increase in the number of people prescribed methadone in Manchester between 1985 and 1994, the number of opiate addicts increased slightly more than three-fold. Addiction specialists are the new Canutes, bidding the tide recede, but without Canute's awareness that the tide did not obey him.) In England and Wales as a whole, there were 9 deaths associated with methadone in 1985; by 1992 there were 115.

There has been an upsurge recently in the United States in deaths associated with methadone, so that in states such as Florida and North Carolina they are more numerous than deaths associated with heroin. The upsurge appears to have been caused largely by the increased number of prescriptions of methadone by doctors for pain, rather than for opiate addiction,; but the drug is being diverted by those who have fooled their doctors into prescribing it into what one might call the usual illicit channels. The doctors are just as easily fooled by people pretending to be in severe pain as by addicts, and with the same results. In 1997, there were 3,832 emergency room attendances caused principally by methadone; in 2001, there were 10,725. In Florida, methadone-related deaths increased 56 percent between 2001 and 2002 alone, from 357 to 556. This gives us no reason to be confident that, if only doctors were liberal enough with methadone prescriptions, large numbers of lives would be saved. Yet the impression is often given in the literature that if only we could get enough methadone into enough people, the social problem of opiate addiction would be solved.

It is certainly possible to reduce the number of deaths associated with methadone by ensuring that it is taken daily under supervision, at a clinic or a pharmacy. In this way, people who are prescribed it are unable to accumulate dangerous (or lucrative) quantities of it. In Glasgow, where it became the official policy to dispense methadone in this fashion, deaths from methadone, which had been rising fast, declined at once by 90 percent, despite a greatly increased number of prescriptions for the drug. In Sheffield, the number of methadone-associated deaths declined, despite a doubling of prescriptions (though the death rate from all opiate deaths doubled at the same time, hardly a public health triumph for methadone treatment).

One might have thought that these experiences would have produced a great effect on the harm-reduction school of thought, and altered practice as a matter of urgency, but one would be mistaken. Methadone continues to be prescribed elsewhere in Britain in the same careless way, with the consequent toll of death, while the United States has moved from tighter to looser prescription, citing Great Britain as a model to be emulated. The failure of harm-reducers to worry very much about the harm they do casts doubt upon their motives, or at least their style of thought.

Even those researchers whose results might be deemed favorable to the prescription of methadone at best damn with faint praise. A recent paper in the journal *Addiction* is entitled "Trends in drug overdose deaths in England and Wales 1993—1998: methadone does not kill more people than heroin." Just imagine a paper in a surgical journal: "Trends in post-operative death after prostatectomy: prostatectomy does not cause more deaths than prostate cancer."

But even this paper, which may be taken to be implicitly supporting the prescription of methadone, purports to show only that the dramatic increase in opiate overdose deaths in England and Wales is not attributable to methadone. The fact remains (and one that is not much emphasized) that heroin was involved in 58 percent of the 3961 fatal poisonings from opiates between 1993 and 1998, while methadone was involved in 49 percent of such poisonings. A harm reduction that consists of not being wholly responsible for an increase in harm is probably better described as a job opportunity.

The New Methadone

Other drugs are on the horizon to do the job that methadone is supposed to do but does so equivocally. Actually, the cure of opiate addiction by the substitution of other drugs has a long history, most famously that of Freud's attempts simultaneously to win world fame for himself by making a startling discovery and to wean his friend and colleague, Dr. von Fleischl-Marxow, from his addiction of morphine by the use of the newly-isolated drug, cocaine. It is true that Fleischl-Marxow stopped taking morphine for a very short time, soon resuming however, but unfortunately was equally soon taking so much cocaine that he suffered its toxic effects, for example the sensation of snakes crawling over his skin. The different drugs that have been suggested as substitutes or adjuncts in the treatment of opiate addiction would be quite sufficient by themselves to fill an entire pharmacopeia. Even Vichy water was said at one time to reduce the craving for opiates in those addicts who were attempting to abstain.

The latest hopeful in the very long line is a drug called buprenorphine. It both stimulates and blockades the opiate receptors in the brain. Widely used in France, it certainly seems a good deal safer than methadone. Since 1996, when it was first used in France, there have been 137 deaths associated with it there (usually when injected and always in conjunction with tranquilizing drugs). Since 60,000 addicts are now under treatment with it, this is not a large number, comparatively speaking, though even its most enthusiastic advocates admit that the number of deaths may be a considerable underestimate.

As far as efficacy is concerned, it is generally believed to be as effective (or as ineffective) as methadone. A trial published in *The New England Journal of Medicine* in 2000 divided 220 addicts into four groups, who received high dose methadone, low dose methadone, buprenorphine, or another long-acting opiate, levomethadyl acetate, respectively. They were followed up for seventeen weeks (not exactly an eternity, or the temporal basis upon which to conclude very much); 73 percent of the high dose methadone patients stayed the course while only 58 percent of the buprenorphine ones did. 28 percent of the high dose methadone patients and 26 percent of the buprenorphine ones had urine samples negative for drugs of abuse, other than those they were prescribed, on twelve consecutive occasions. Perhaps I am too perfectionist, but this does not seem much of a therapeutic triumph to me, nor one that is likely to translate into great social improvement even when extrapolated to thousands of patients.

Buprenorphine has the potential for abuse and diversion on to the open market. In Finland, for example, it is already one of the favored drugs of abuse, and is smuggled from France to that end. A survey conducted in France found that between one in six and one in seven people prescribed the drug had used it for injection. The American Food and Drug Administration's system for recording adverse events connected with drugs reveals a surprisingly high number of side-effects reported with buprenorphine, many of them caused when patients crush the tablet and either dissolve the powder for injection or inhale it through their nose: suggesting that, when it is widely prescribed in America, it might give rise to numerous problems.

Buprenorphine is given in tablets that dissolve under the tongue, because it is poorly absorbed from the gut (the reason it is comparatively safe in oral overdose). One small indication, however, that buprenorphine has potential as a drug of abuse is the fact that the sublingual tablets that are sometimes prescribed in the prison in which I work are known as "furries" when they are removed from under the tongue before they have fully dissolved and passed on to someone else. By their argot shall ye know them. Incidentally, this practice demonstrates that the basis on which the tablet is prescribed in the first place—that withdrawal is intolerable—is false, for if it were intolerable no one would be willing to forego the relief it provided.

At best, then, buprenorphine is likely to be safer than methadone, and to that extent it is more likely actually to reduce harm than methadone. And it is certainly true that in France, the sudden, explosive increase in the prescription of buprenorphine, legalized in 1996, has coincided with a dramatic reduction in the numbers of deaths from poisoning by opiates. In fact, this reduction is too great to be attributable to the prescription alone: while an estimated third of opiate addicts in France have received such a prescription, deaths have declined by three-quarters. Some other factor, therefore, must also be involved. *Post hoc* is not *propter hoc*.

In all probability, we are going through the honeymoon period that often follows the introduction of a new drug that appears to have many and various advantages and no disadvantages. When methadone was first introduced as a treatment for heroin addiction, it resulted in near-miraculous figures of improvement in the hands of those who discovered or developed this use. Methadone was the buprenorphine of its day. Only years later did its drawbacks, its very considerable drawbacks, become clear (if often wilfully ignored). I thus make a prediction, which, however, might, of course, be disproved with the passage of time: that in a few years there will be a controversy as to the efficacy and safety of buprenorphine. In the meantime, it will have been dispensed like confetti at a wedding.

Finally, the logic on which it is prescribed is the same as that upon which methadone is prescribed, which is faulty even if the drug itself proves once and for all to be safer.

Summary

It is now time to summarize. There is a standard view of heroin addiction that is wrong in almost all its particulars. Heroin hooks no one: it takes effort and determination to reach a stage of addiction, complete with all its sequelae. Withdrawal from heroin is not medically serious or even horribly unpleasant, except in the fevered imagination of those who have been encouraged to think that it is. Heroin addiction does not drive people into crime, as a billiard cue drives a billiard ball before it: it would be truer to say that a criminal disposition drives people to heroin. It is not true that once addicted, a person is a slave to the drug, or a Haitian zombie, with no power whatever to make decisions for himself: millions of people have abandoned opiate addiction when they have sufficiently strong motives to do so. It therefore follows that professional help is not necessary for a person to give up. It is not true that the provision of ever more services for drug addicts has been accompanied by a decrease in drug addiction or in any of the social problems associated with it. On the contrary, the social pathology connected with heroin addiction, or of which it is itself a manifestation, has increased regardless of the services provided for addicts, and indeed it is more plausible to say that such services have resulted in an increase rather than a decrease in the problems to which they are ostensibly the solution. It is not true that any improvement in the social functioning of addicts given replacement therapy (the predominant form of therapy) is necessarily accompanied by an improvement in society in general. This is false logic, and it is easy to see why. If so, then no treatment, at least of a quasi-medical nature, will ever do the things we want it to do. It is more likely to spread the problem than to solve it.

When I ask prisoners whether they have any medical problems and they reply, "Heroin addiction," I in turn reply that heroin addiction is not a medical problem. Although they are not generally the most intellectually gifted or sophisticated of people, they understand precisely what I mean, even though my remark is in a sense cryptic and misses out all of the premises upon which it is based. Many of them smile, as if caught out in something; many of them say, "Yes, I know." The game is up.

II

The Literature of Exaggeration and Self-Dramatization

But oh! That deep romantic chasm which slanted
Down the green hill athwart a cedarn cover!
A savage place! As holy and enchanted
As e'er beneath a waning moon was haunted
By woman wailing for her demon-lover!

—Samuel Taylor Coleridge,
"Kubla Khan"

In modern society the main cause of drug addiction, apart from the fact that many people have nothing to live for, is a literary tradition of romantic claptrap, started by Coleridge and De Quincey, and continued without serious interruption ever since. It received a new lease of life in the 1960s, when countercultural figures proclaimed the mind-expanding properties of illicit drugs, an illusion, as Harvey Mansfield put it, so pathetic that one can hardly credit that it was once held. This claptrap is the main source of popular and medical misconceptions on the subject.

The Literary Tradition: Evasiveness

Romantic claptrap invests intoxication by opiates with a philosophical significance beyond mere self-indulgence. The idea is that an addled brain is capable of insights into the nature of existence deeper than those produced by the clearest mind. It also encourages people to suppose that rebellion against society, in the form of such intoxication, is a good in itself, and is self-justifying, no matter what is being rebelled against or what the consequences might be, personal or social. It elevates feeling and intuition above knowledge and thought in the pantheon of human desiderata. It invests the personal pettiness of addiction with the aura of titanic and tormenting struggles against mighty forces, while at the same time implying that there is a connection between opiates, talent, creativity and genius. It encourages histrionic self-dramatization, to the detriment of real character.

De Quincey was most insistent, in the second and much expanded edition of his *Confessions,* that his use of laudanum had nothing whatever to do with self-indulgence, though in the process he mounts a defense of self-indulgence, asking why, if it is permissible in the case of alcohol, it is not permissible in the case of opium: the question asked by libertarian theorists and practicing reprobates ever since. De Quincey's verbiage soon raises smokescreens which it is almost impossible for the average reader—that is to say, the reader who is merely curious—to penetrate. His very prose style suggests an inveterate tendency to self-indulgence: indeed, at one point he says "my way of writing is rather to think aloud and follow my own humors than much to consider who is listening to me," indicating a less than total commitment to consecutive thought.

De Quincey starts his second edition thus:

> I have often been asked—how it was, and through what series of steps, that I became an opium-eater. Was it gradually, tentatively, mistrustingly, as one goes down a shelving beach into a deepening sea, and with a knowledge from the first of the dangers lying on that path; half-courting those dangers, in fact, while seeming to defy them? Or was it, secondly, in pure ignorance of such dangers, under the misleadings of mercenary fraud? ... Thirdly, and lastly, was it (*Yes*, by passionate anticipation, I answer, before the question is finished)—was it on a sudden, overmastering impulse derived from bodily anguish?

After a disquisition of the false differences sometimes urged between his case and Coleridge's, Coleridge supposedly having taken opium solely for illness and De Quincey for pleasure, he says:

> Most truly I have told the reader, that not any search after pleas-
> ure, but mere extremity of pain from rheumatic toothache—this
> and nothing else it was that first drove me to the use of opium....
> In this stage of the suffering, formed and perfect, I was thrown
> passively upon chance advice, and therefore, by a natural conse-
> quence, upon opium—that being the one sole anodyne that is
> almost notoriously such, and which in that great function is uni-
> versally appreciated.

In the first edition of his work, De Quincey says that he first
took opium in order to soothe his stomach, which (he says) was
disordered by experiences in his youth, and which he then describes
in irrelevant, and therefore obfuscating, detail. Opium, he says,
was the only effective relief for it, which is why he continued to
take it. There is nothing of toothache in the first edition to blame
the commencement of his addiction on; thus De Quincey either
cannot remember, or is lying about, why he first took opium,
inaugurating a tradition of evasion that has continued ever since,
and that now manifests itself in self-exculpating tales of the
omnipresence of heroin in the social environment, or the malign
influence of unsuitable friends.

Having defended the theoretical or philosophical permissi-
bility of self-indulgence in opium, of its use for mere pleasure, De
Quincey then goes on to disparage Coleridge's use of opium for
precisely the reason that Coleridge had once disparaged De
Quincey's: its self-indulgence. Coleridge claimed that he used
opium only to relieve his rheumatic pains, which De Quincey then
exposes as the merest self-deception:

> Rheumatism, he says, drove him to opium. Very well; but with
> proper medical treatment the rheumatism would soon have ceased;
> or even, without medical treatment, under the ordinary oscilla-
> tions of natural causes. And when the pain ceased, then the opium
> should have ceased. Why did it not? Because Coleridge had come
> to taste the genial pleasure of opium .... It is really memorable in
> the annals of human self-deceptions, that Coleridge could have
> held such language in the face of the facts.

I suppose that self-deception could be defined as untruth
that one easily recognizes as such when uttered by another, but

unrecognized (though of course not unrecognizable) when uttered by oneself. And here really is a case of the pot calling the kettle black.

I have already quoted De Quincey to the effect that for many years he took laudanum only on Saturday nights. He even states that he took it so infrequently in order that it might continue to have its full psychological effect upon him, which suggests that he was not so unacquainted with the phenomenon of physiological tolerance as he makes out, and that in fact he was aware of at least some of the addictive properties (half-courting those dangers, in fact, while seeming to defy them) of opium when he first set out on taking it.

And this awareness, or awareness half-denied, continues to the present day. The vast majority of opiate addicts in contemporary societies are not ignorant of the addictive properties of opiates before they ever take these drugs for the first, second, and nth time. Even if governments had not extensively propagandized on this subject, only the deaf and blind could have remained in ignorance. Even the excuse that "I thought it could never happen to me" is feeble and implausible, in view of the numbers of addicts every person who addicts himself knows before he does so.

The Literary Tradition: Wisdom by Intoxication

Saturday nights were the nights when De Quincey attended the opera.

> Now opium, by greatly increasing the activity of the mind generally, increases ... that particular mode of its activity by which we are able to construct out of the raw material of organic sound an elaborate intellectual pleasure ...; it is sufficient to say, that a chorus ... displayed before me ... the whole of my past life ... and its passions exalted, spiritualized, and sublimed.

This is high flown, no doubt, but at the very least it is clear we are now a long way from abdominal discomfort or toothache and the relief of the pain thereof. De Quincey believed that opium propelled him into spiritual regions inaccessible by other routes. De Quincey spotted Coleridge's self-deceptions all right; but he was completely blind to his own.

A superior appreciation of, or at least response to, music was not the only advantage or pleasure of opium. In his comparison of opium with alcohol, De Quincey ascribes to opium various desirable effects:

> Opium ... introduces amongst [the mental faculties] the most exquisite order, legislation, and harmony .... [O]pium communicates serenity and equipoise to all the faculties, active or passive .... [O]pium ... gives an expansion to the heart and the benevolent affections .... [T]he expansion of the beniger feelings, incident to opium, is no febrile access, but a healthy restoration to that state which the mind would naturally recover upon the removal of any deep-seated irritation of pain that had disturbed and quarrelled with the impulses of a heart originally just and good .... [O]pium always seems to compose what had been agitated, and to concentrate what had been distracted.... [T]he opium eater ... feels that the diviner part of his nature is paramount; that is, the moral affections are in a state of cloudless serenity; and over all is the great light of the majestic intellect.

Gosh! Opium not only calms you down while sharpening your faculties and honing your intelligence, but makes you a better, kinder person. No pharmaceutical purveyor of an antidepressant ever bid up his product higher than that. Take but a little heroin, therefore, and your intellect will be majestic. Your thoughts will be coherent, your powers of mental synthesis unparalleled. You will recover the pristine, pre-social beauty of the human character of which Rousseau speaks so eloquently. A drunk is a drunk, but a heroin addict is a philosopher.

According to De Quincey, he who takes opiates is privileged to experience a state of mind of exquisite sensitivity, unknown to the rest of us:

> markets and theatres are not the appropriate haunts of the opium-eater, when in the divinest state incident to his enjoyment. In that state, crowds become an oppression to him; music even, too sensual and gross. He naturally seeks solitude and silence, an indispensable condition of those trances, or profoundest reveries, which are the crown and consummation of what opium can do for human nature.

De Quincey takes it for granted that opium can do a lot for human nature.

Unfortunately, as De Quincey acknowledges grandiloquently and hyperbolically (we shall come to that in due course), opium has its pains as well as its pleasures. But even the pains are an assurance of the worth of him who suffers them, according to De Quincey. At the end of *Suspiria de profundis,* he says:

> Pain driven to agony, or grief driven to frenzy, is essential to the ventilation of profound natures.

Suffering is the precondition of profundity: we see here a glimpse of the romantic underpinning of the modern taste for self-destruction, which is now a mass phenomenon. For when suffering will not come to you, you must go to it, at least if you want to be considered profound. And by an error of logic that is so common as to be almost universal, people suppose that if persons of a profound nature need suffering to bring out their profundity, then the fact of suffering, however caused, is itself proof of profundity. He who has not suffered the pains of opium or heroin (there can be no greater, of course) is therefore not a profound person, but someone who has merely skated easily over the surface of life.

Of course, De Quincey has already given abundant evidence of his liability to exaggerate the significance of quite banal experiences, a characteristic that he shared with Coleridge, who had it in spades, as it were. For example, De Quincey describes a period of his life when, as a hungry and homeless youth in London, he is befriended by a prostitute called Ann. He tells us how Ann once saved his life. They were sitting together on the steps of a house:

> I had been leaning my head against her bosom; and all at once I sank from her arms and fell backwards on the steps. From the sensations I then had, I felt an inner conviction of the liveliest kind that without some powerful and reviving stimulant, I should either have died on the spot—or should at least have sunk to a point of exhaustion from which all re-ascent under my friendless circumstances would soon have become hopeless. Then it was, at this crisis of my fate, that my poor orphan companion—who had herself

met with little but injuries in this world—stretched out a saving hand to me.

And what did she do to save De Quincey's life? She bought him a glass of port wine and spices, whereof he drank and continued to live. Indeed, the port had "an instantaneous power of restoration."

The sheer physiological implausibility of a glass of port wine (even with spices) saving anyone's life—and elsewhere in the book, De Quincey calls Ann his "saviour," so he meant it quite literally—has never caused anyone to doubt the veracity or verisimilitude of De Quincey's account, or rather accounts, of himself. But a man given to such hyperbole is scarcely the reliable guide to physiology or even to his own experience that he has been taken ever since to be by gullible litterateurs and medical men alike. In other words, De Quincey inaugurated the gross inflation of personal experience that continues to characterize opiate addicts, who to this day are to be found shamelessly rolling in agony when they do not receive what they want, even in the midst of people in hospital with real cause for agony, generally borne with dignity and fortitude. Any doctor who has had to deal, as I have had to do on so many occasions, with this false and histrionic agony will have experienced an inner tension caused by the need to suppress irritation at such patent dishonesty and to retain a professional calm. One easy way to relieve this tension is to assume that all expressions of distress indicate real distress of one kind or other; and simulaneously to hold this truth to be self-evident, that all distresses are created equal. Such a seemingly "understanding" view is naive in its human psychology, as any child who has thrown a tantrum and subsequently reflected upon its real cause would be able to tell you, but it is comforting to those who want urgently to end emotional blackmail by the easiest expedient, which is to give in to it.

On De Quincey's account, the opiate habitué has had experiences that set him apart from (and higher, though also lower, than) the rest of the human race. And there is very little doubt that running through much of the opium and opiate literature that succeeds De Quincey, there is a strong feeling of the intellectual, moral and spiritual superiority of the opiate-experienced.

Opium is often said to give people insights unavailable to those too conventional, too respectable or too frightened to try. It is true that De Quincey at one point says that if a man's thoughts when not taking opium are of oxen, then it is of oxen that he will dream when he does take opium. But everything else he says suggests that opium (and, *a fortiori*, the pure compounds derived from it) sharpens and deepens the mental faculties and gives depth both to thoughts and sensations. But by its fruits shall you know the philosophical enlightenment of opiate addiction. A hundred years after De Quincey published his book, a British officer in Burma, Captain H. H. Robinson, also took to opium and believed that, in his opium-befuddled trances, he achieved a high degree of philosophical insight. His book—called *A Modern De Quincey,* published in 1942—describes how one day he steeled himself to write down the truth vouchsafed to him in this state, that he believed had penetrated to the essence of human existence. "The banana is great," he wrote, "but the banana skin is greater." Though Captain Robinson repeats the mythological horrors of withdrawal, he is at least disarmingly frank about the banality of opium thoughts. I have heard a lot of addicts speak under the influence of their drug, and even as they are just coming round from a coma induced by an overdose, and I have yet to hear from them a single arresting thought, at least in propositional form.

And yet the myth that opiates open a path to wisdom and higher knowledge has enjoyed a more or less continuous vogue ever since De Quincey wrote. I give examples of this in the appendix.

The Literary Tradition: Wisdom and Transcendent Knowledge at a Stroke

The desire that there should be a short-cut to the deepest knowledge and wisdom is one that we all share. Because we do not understand the nature of consciousness, we have no understanding of where our own ideas come from, and it is a short step from this ignorance to the supposition that strokes of genius can arrive without effort on the part of those having them. Mozart is said to have taken dictation from God, and is popularly depicted (in the play and film *Amadeus,* for example), as being a posturing ninny who just happened to have been born with a prodigious gift. No one could possibly doubt that he was born with a prodigious gift, of course, but Mozart was very hard-working too, and in his famous letter to Haydn, in which he dedicated his six quartets to the great master, he alludes to the close and detailed study he had given to the form, which clearly did not well up in him like water from a hot spring. Similarly, Dostoyevsky, misled I think by the ecstatic auras of his epileptic fits, believed that redemptive remorse and insight into the divine nature of things could arrive suddenly, almost unbidden, without effort. The idea that psychoactive drugs, opiates not least among them, might lead to profundity and creativity is not without cognate notions.

For myself, I think that good evidence for the proposition that heroin and other opiates powerfully stimulate the intellectual, creative or spiritual faculties of man needs to be offered. Jack Gelber's play *The Connection*, from which I quote in the appendix, implies a connection between heroin and creativity by making use of jazz musicians who improvise for long periods throughout it (it would hardly be a full-length play otherwise). As is well known, many famous jazz musicians were addicted to heroin, and the implication in Gelber's play is that heroin addiction is causally related to their creativity.

The idea that opiates stimulate the imagination and are therefore an aid to creativity goes back to the Romantics and even a little before. The founder of American psychiatry, and signatory of the Declaration of Independence, Benjamin Rush, once wrote of a case of a young man who informed him that, when he took his habitual opium, "his intellects were more brilliant, his language more eloquent, and his talent for writing more easy, than in the former and healthy period of his life." (This was published eighteen years before the first edition of De Quincey's *Confessions.*)

There is little doubt that a connection between opiate addiction and creativity has insinuated itself into popular consciousness. De Quincey attributed his brilliant dreams (which, more properly, are his brilliant reports of his dreams) to the effects of opium. And intense dreams are sometimes the midwives of great work, or so it is believed. Robert Louis Stevenson's *The Strange*

Case of Doctor Jekyll and Mr. Hyde came to him in a dream (at least the story did, if not the complete version), as did, allegedly, the structure of the benzene ring to the German chemist Frederick August Kekule, who said that he dreamed of a snake swallowing its own tail. If opiates stimulate dreams, and dreams stimulate creativity, then opiates are an aid to the creative.

Dickens took this up, or swallowed whole, the notion of opium as a stimulant of dreams in the opening page of his last book, *The Mystery of Edwin Drood*, in which Mr. Jasper is lying in an opium den in the city of whose cathedral he is lay precentor:

> An ancient English Cathedral Tower? How can the ancient English Cathedral be here! The well-known massive grey square tower of its old Cathedral? How can that be here! There is no spike of rusty iron in the air, between the eye and it, from any point of the real prospect. What is this spike that intervenes, and who has set it up? Maybe, it is set up by the Sultan's orders for the impaling of a horde of Turkish robbers, one by one. It is so, for cymbals clash, and the Sultan goes by to his palace in long procession. Ten thousand scimitars flash in the sunlight, and thrice ten thousand dancing-girls strew flowers. Then, follow white elephants caparisoned in countless gorgeous colors, and infinite in numbers and attendants. Still, the Cathedral Tower rises in the background, where it cannot be, and still no writhing figure is on the grim spike. Stay! Is the spike so low a thing as the rusty spike on the top of a post of an old bedstead that has tumbled all awry?

It isn't very difficult to guess where Dickens derived either his idea or imagery from. Coleridge told the story of how the poem "Kubla Khan" came to him, and Dickens must have known both the poem and the story. This is Coleridge's account in his preface to the poem of how he came to compose it:

> In the summer of the year 1797, the Author, then in ill health, had retired to a lonely farm-house between Porlock and Linton, on the Exmoor confines of Somerset and Devonshire. In consequence of a slight indisposition, an anodyne had been prescribed, from the effects of which he fell asleep in his chair at the moment that he was reading the following sentence, or words of the same substance, in "Purchas's Pilgrimage": "Here the Khan Kubla commanded a palace to be built, and a stately garden thereunto. And

thus ten miles of fertile ground were inclosed with a wall." The Author continued for about three hours in a profound sleep, at least of the external senses, during which time he has the most vivid confidence, that he could not have composed less than from two to three hundred lines; if that indeed can be called composition in which all the images rose up before him as *things*, with a parallel production of the correspondent expressions, without any sensation or consciousness of effort. On awaking he appeared to himself to have a distinct recollection of the whole, and taking his pen, ink, and paper, instantly and eagerly wrote down the lines that are here preserved.

Influential literary critics and scholars have accepted this version of the origin of the poem, though some of Coleridge's own contemporaries doubted it, Robert Southey, for example, believing that Coleridge only dreamt that he dreamed Kubla Khan. Coleridge was notoriously inexact when it came to facts, especially about his own life, believing rather in a higher, poetic truth. But there is little doubt that his account, however much or often refuted by scholars subsequently, has entered the mythology of opium (and therefore opiates) as an aid to the expression of genius. The fact that Coleridge had already written "The Ancient Mariner," and that it has been conclusively proved, insofar as such things can be conclusively proved, that it was not composed under the influence of opium, and that therefore Coleridge's poetic gifts did not require opium for their expression, has not affected the myth, which is virtually indestructible. Nor does anyone wonder whether, even if it were true that his two great poems were the product of opium consumption, the light would be worth the candle. Two poems, one might have thought, however great they are, is not very much to show for all the devastation wrought upon people's lives by the habitual use of opiates.

Ah! But other writers were opiate addicts! Wilkie Collins is said to have written several chapters—some of the most important ones—of *The Moonstone*, while in an opiate haze (he, too, was an addict), scarcely conscious of what he did. And the English poets George Crabbe and Francis Thompson were likewise addicts. And a whole theory of the beneficial effects of opium has been raised upon these slight foundations, a theory which I suspect has eventually had a great, if indefinable effect upon popular thought on the matter. (Interestingly, the great propagandist for the emancipation of slaves and the termination of the Atlantic slave trade, William Wilberforce, was an opiate addict till the end of his life, but no one, so far as I know, has yet proposed that his activities were the consequence of his addiction.)

In 1934, long before he became a well-known literary critic, a young scholar called M. H. Abrams published a little book that, he said, started as a sophomore essay at Harvard, and certainly it bears the stigmata of its origin: which, however, is not to say that it was without influence. It has been reprinted at least twice. The book was entitled *The Milk of Paradise,* and is subtitled *The Effect of Opium Visions on the Works of De Quincey, Crabbe, Francis Thompson and Coleridge.* (The "milk of Paradise" appears in a line in "Kubla Khan.") The burden of this book is as follows:

> The great gift of opium to these men was access to a new world as different from this as Mars may be; and one which ordinary mortals, hindered by terrestrial conceptions, can never, from mere description, quite comprehend. It is a world of twisted, exquisite experience, sensuous and intellectual; of "music like a perfume," and "sweet light golden with audible odors exquisite," where color is a symphony, and one can hear the walk of an insect on the ground, the bruising of a flower. Above all, in this enchanted land man is freed at last from those petty bonds upon which Kant insists: space and time. Space is amplified to such proportions that, to writer after writer, "infinity" is the only word adequate to compass it. More striking still, man escapes at last from the life of transiency lamented by poets since time immemorial, and approaches immortality as closely as he ever can in this world; for he experiences, almost literally, eternity.

Phew! Not bad for a drug! One wonders how anyone—Shakespeare, for example—could have got by without it. The mystic enlightenment brought about by opiates is not so very different from what the Buddha experienced, at least as described by Professor R. C. Zaehner, in his book *Drugs, Mysticism and Make-believe:*

> the Buddha's own experience of what the Buddhists call "enlightenment"—or more literally "awakening"—which means, among

other things, the conquest of death by transcending everything that binds us to this world of space and time.

One might also cite here William James' conclusions having inhaled nitrous oxide, or laughing gas:

> One conclusion was forced upon my mind at that time, and my impression of its truth has ever remained unshaken. It is that our normal waking consciousness, rational consciousness as we call it, is but one special type of consciousness, whilst all about it, parted from it by the filmiest of screens, there lie potential forms of consciousness entirely different. We may go through life without suspecting their existence; but apply the requisite stimulus, and at a touch they are there in all their completeness, definite types of mentality which probably somewhere have their field of application and adaptation.

This is not very far from De Quincey's remark in the *Confessions,* "I shall be charged with mysticism," or indeed from his assertion that an elixir of wisdom was to be found in a bottle. And with authorities such as these, who is a poor slum-dweller to argue, especially when his chances of reaching enlightenment any other way are severely circumscribed by lack of education, culture and possibly intelligence? Is it any surprise that many addicts have told me that they feel that, under the influence of heroin, they have reached a deeper level of understanding than any other known to them, and that I am not in a position to deny it because—in the cant phrase of our times—I haven't been there?

Besides, we live in a democratic, not to say demotic, age: so why should the beneficial, not to say miraculous, effects of opium (and opiates) be confined to "these men," "the writer after writer" (four, actually, or five if one counts Arthur Symons, who coined the phrases "music like a perfume" and "sweet light golden with audible odors exquisite") who were able to eternalize themselves by means of them, according to M. H. Abrams? Why should the devil have all the best tunes, and the poets all the best drugs? (De Quincey was not strictly a poet, but his prose was poetic, in the sense of being long-winded and saying things that were not strictly true.) If men of genius take opiates, does it not follow that taking opiates will make us men of genius? Perhaps it does not follow in strict logic, but psychologically it follows. Besides, if opium (and opiates) offered up vistas "measureless to man" to men like Coleridge and De Quincey, why should they not do so for us? Is it not an article of faith (not least among modern educationists) that, lurking in the brain or soul of every man, there is a deep well of creativity waiting to be tapped?

To establish beyond doubt that opium and opiates were mid-wives to works of genius and to superhuman states of mind would require more than a few anecdotes about a handful of poets, some being not as great as all that. It would require a statistical comparison of people of equal talent, some of whom, unbeknown to them, took opiates, and the rest of whom, equally unbeknown to them, did not. (If the experimental subjects knew either that they were or were not taking opiates, their performance might be affected other than pharmacologically, the reputation of opiates for stimulating the imagination being what it is.) Needless to say, such an experiment could never actually be carried out, so we will never have a definitive answer.

Of course, a definitively negative answer to the question of whether opiates stimulate imaginative genius cannot be given either. But common sense informs us that the worthwhile cultural products of millions of addicts have been exiguous, to say the least, and that a biographical examination of the lives of Baudelaire, Coleridge, and De Quincey (the best advertisements for opiates, after all) leads us to the conclusion that opiates harmed rather than stimulated their talents. De Quincey and Coleridge both had vast philosophical ambitions, but never completed an important work of philosophy, De Quincey in particular suffering long fallow periods: and I suspect that their opiate addiction may have been a means to disguise from themselves the limitations of their philosophical abilities. As for Baudelaire, his notorious procrastination and his relatively small output might well be attributable to his opiate addiction: the world might have had more of his poems, not less great than those he actually wrote, had he not taken opium.

The kind of romantic nonsense that sees opiates as an aid to genius and enlightenment has, of course, been repeated in full with regard to other drugs such as cannabis, mescalin, and lysergic acid. But the attitude to opium and opiates was its model or template, and added nothing new from the doctrinal point of view.

The Literary Tradition: The Romance of Negation

There is one other romantic attraction of opiates: and that is to the antinomian turn of mind. This turn of mind has become much more common with the general rise of self-importance, which is a corollary of democracy: and in an age of celebrity, everyone feels obliged to leave his mark on the world, or else feel an intolerable wound to his ego. It is often rather difficult to make a mark on the world in a positive way, by the invention of something, for example, or by genuine scholarship or artistic creation, so that all that remains for the person who wishes to make his mark is opposition, bloody-mindedness, destruction and the breaking of taboos (by which is often meant perfectly reasonable social prohibitions of the kind upon which the preservation of civilization depends).

Let us turn again to the case of William Burroughs, that walking, living, breathing compendium of psychopathology. In his first, highly autobiographical book *Junkie* he says that "Kick (i.e. of heroin) is seeing things from a special angle. Kick is momentary freedom from the claims of the aging, cautious, nagging, frightened flesh." Laws for the suppression of opiate consumption are "police state legislation penalizing a state of being:" a state of being that, when viewed through the lens of moral relativism, is as "valid" as any other. (Moral relativism is always relative, of course: police state legislation is evil incarnate, and poor innocent William Burroughs "saw my chance of escaping conviction dwindle as the anti-junk feeling mounted to a paranoid obsession, like anti-Semitism under the Nazis." I think the comparison between himself and victims of the extermination camps requires no comment.) So Burroughs also had a quasi-philosophical reason, or rationalization, for taking heroin, even if at other times he states that, after a short time, the only reason to take heroin is to avoid the pains of withdrawal ("Junk takes everything and gives nothing but insurance against junk sickness"): namely, it gives you a special "angle" and puts you in a different way of being, that are not available to the abstainer, who—by implication—is missing something valuable.

But there is more to Burroughs' philosophy, to give it a charitable name, than that. As we have seen, he was twelve years old when he read a book by a petty criminal, Jack Black, entitled *You Can't Win* that impressed him very deeply. Over sixty years later, he wrote an introduction to a republication of the book. He wrote:

> Stultified and confined by middle-class St. Louis mores, I was fascinated by this glimpse of an underworld of seedy rooming houses, pool parlors, cat houses and opium dens, of bull pens and cat burglars and hobo jungles. I learned of good bums and thieves . . . with a code of conduct that made more sense to me than the arbitrary, hypocritical rules that were taken for granted as being "right" by my peers.

It evidently didn't occur to Burroughs that, man being a fallen creature, any demanding code of rules would be broken by everyone who claimed to uphold them, you and me included, and that the only way to avoid hypocrisy altogether was to have no rules whatever beyond "Do what you feel like." Besides, Burroughs himself was no mean hypocrite: his alleged contempt for the "system" and for his bourgeois parents did not in the least prevent him accepting a monetary allowance from them, which permitted him to live as a parasite on the work of others, for many years. And let us pass over in silence the state of terribly arrested intellectual development that made the moral effect of a book read when twelve years old exactly the same when re-read as a seventy-two years old.

Burroughs goes on to write:

> Re-reading the book fifty years later, I felt a deep nostalgia for a way of life that is gone forever.

What exactly is it that makes Burroughs eyes mist over with filmy tears of sentiment? "Scenes and characters," he says, "emerge from the pages, bathed in the light of past times." But what scenes, what characters? This is the scene and these are the characters that he chooses in order to remind us of the bittersweet passage of time, whose arrow flies in one direction only, and that arouses so powerful a nostalgia in him:

> This young gay cat starts bad-mouthing Salt Chunk Mary and old George—a railriding safecracker with two fingers missing from crimping blasting caps—says to him: "You were a good bum, but you're dog meat now," and shot him four times across the fire at a hobo jungle, and I could feel the slugs hit him. He fell down with his hair in the fire. Turns out Salt Chunk Mary is George's sister. Sister or not, the gay cat was out of line to talk against a women like Salt Chunk Mary.

One might have thought that this was not altogether a tactful choice of illustrative incident for a man who had shot his wife dead, allegedly accidentally, but more likely accidentally-on-purpose, and had never been penalized for it beyond a fine (of course paid by his hypocritical, inauthentic parents). Aesthetic considerations aside, however, his admiration for what this passage represents bespeaks a Gnostic, or even a Satanic, reversal of values. Milton's Satan says, as he is expelled from heaven:

> So farewell Hope, and with Hope farewell Fear,
> Farewell Remorse: all Good to me is lost;
> Evil be thou my Good.

And Evil was Burroughs' good, once he had expelled himself from the paradise of American bourgeoisie.

The weekend before I wrote this, I happened to be called in to the prison in which I work as a doctor. When I refused to prescribe certain drugs for a prisoner who wanted them (he was in prison for, among other things, breaking the fingers of old women in his haste to remove their rings from them), on the reasonable grounds that I thought there was no medical indication for such drugs, he threatened to kill me and called my mother a whore. Had I reacted like George in defense of a women of whom it was "out of line" to talk in this fashion, and killed him, Burroughs would have lost no time in condemning me; but had the prisoner actually succeeded in killing me as he threatened, he would no doubt have turned my death into an amusing anecdote about which it would be permissible and even *de rigueur* to be nostalgic a few years later. That is because in Burroughs' view a man who breaks the fingers of old women while robbing them is a good man, while a doctor trying to perform his duty is, *ex offi-cio* as it were, a bad one.

This extraordinary reversal of values is confirmed by Burroughs' evident response to Jack Black's description of junkies: "Their bony arms were gray, like pieces of petrified wood. The skin was pocked with marks, mottled and scarred from the repeated, hourly stabbing of the needle. Their shirtsleeves were encrusted with the blood from the many punctures." Black's description has the merit of being truthful, and would put most people off addiction rather than attract them to it. But it seems to have had the reverse effect on Burroughs, for whom only the ugly, vicious, degraded, and repellent were truly authentic, and for whom only the truly authentic was worth aiming for. As it happens, it is not very difficult to be repellent: everyone can manage it if he tries—success is virtually guaranteed.

This modern Gnostic attitude, which is the ego's revolt against the frustrating but inevitable demands of society, is not confined to Burroughs by any means. One might almost call it the dominant literary conceit of the twentieth century, and it is purely Romantic in inspiration. You have only to think of Norman Mailer's exhortation to us to cultivate our inner psychopath and live solely for the moment, published in the same year as Burroughs' *Naked Lunch,* to understand the lengths to which such dishonest romantic claptrap may go. And while Romanticism started as a movement among poets and litterateurs, in a society that took human hierarchy for granted, accepting that certain exquisite experiences were beyond the reach of the common herd, modern romanticism has accepted *in toto* the democratic supposition that all men are created equal, and therefore have the right to equal access to the spheres of existence allegedly opened up by the consumption of drugs, opiates not least among them.

The hundreds of young prisoners whom I saw who took heroin were perfectly well aware before they ever took it of the connection between criminality and heroin. Far from deterring them, it was one of the things that attracted them to the drug in the first place.

The Literary Tradition: Personal Experience
as a Source of Infallible Knowledge

Having successfully insinuated that the habitual consumption of opiates is of philosophical significance for those who take it, the litterateurs go on to suggest that personal experience is the most important, indeed the only, source of knowledge. De Quincey started this particular ball rolling with regard to opium, in a famous passage in his *Confessions*:

> This is the doctrine of the true church on the subject of opium: of which church I acknowledge myself to be the only member—the alpha and the omega: but then it is to be recollected, that I speak from the ground of a large and profound personal experience: whereas most of the un- scientific authors who have all treated of opium, and even those who have written expressly on the materia medica, make it evident, from the horror they express of it, that their experimental knowledge of its action is none at all.

By "experimental knowledge" De Quincy means, of course, personal experience, the source of his own papal infallibility. And this is a cry that has rung down the ages. No one can speak of drugs in an authoritative fashion unless he has partaken of them himself. In my edition of *Junkie,* there is a glossary of terms that might not have been familiar to the average American reader of the time, including of the word "hip":

> Someone who knows the score. Someone who understands "jive talk." Someone who is "with it." The expression is not subject to definition because, if you don't "dig" what it means, no one can ever tell you.

Such is the doctrine of the true church on the subject of hip. You have to experience it to know what it is, and no one can speak of it who has not tried it.

"No one knows what junk is," writes Burroughs, "until he is junk sick."

In effect, I hear this from addicts very frequently. If I tell them that withdrawal from opiates is not, medically speaking, a serious condition, they reply that I cannot possibly know this, since I have never experienced it myself. In other words, there is no other way of knowing whether a condition is serious or not than by personal experience of it.

This is not only a highly irrationalist theory, one that would make all scientific medicine impossible, but it is also deeply dishonest in its application. The addict who says that the doctor who has not experienced withdrawal for himself cannot know that is not medically serious would not apply the same criterion to any other condition. If a doctor were to tell him, for example, that a sub-conjunctival haemorrhage, while it looks dramatic, is not serious, he would not reply, "How do you know? Have you ever had one yourself?" Nor would anyone dispute a doctor's word if he said that cerebral malaria was a medical emergency, though he had never suffered from it in his life.

I do not mean, of course, to deny the value of personal experience: it is what most of us live for, in one form or another. Nor do I deny that accounts of personal experience are of immense importance to doctors. Much, though not all, diagnosis starts with the patient's account of what he has experienced. A doctor who never listened to what his patient had to say on the matter of personal experience would not get very far. But likewise, a doctor who believed every word his patients said, as a matter of principle, and never attempted to confirm their story against other sources of information, would be very easy to fool, and in not a few cases would end up doing his patients harm rather than good. Denial of what is the case, and assertion of what is not the case, are after all rather common human failings. Personal experience itself, moreover, is subject to a lot of variables: not long ago in a ward in my hospital, a woman suffering from (or perhaps I should say enjoying) mania ran up and down the ward, screaming for joy and laughing uproariously, though she had a severely broken ankle that would have caused anyone else to cry out in pain and remain severely still. Her lack of complaint did not mean that her ankle was any the less in need of treatment, of course. Suffice it to say that he is not most in need of assistance who shouts the loudest, nor was De Quincey in so uniquely privileged a position with regard to his own situation that we must all accept what he said without criticism, or without testing it against other sources of knowledge. Yet this, in essence, is the demand of his addict-followers and disciples down to the present day. And that, no doubt, is why so many addicts have written their memoirs *à la* De Quincey, to make sure that his message, however wrong, is never lost to the world.

The Literary Tradition: The Horrors of Withdrawal and the Agonies of Abstention

And, of course, a very important part of the Romantic message is the insufferable agony of addiction. Only if the agony of withdrawal were insufferable could the addict be altogether absolved of the heinous charge of self-indulgence. Furthermore, in order to add to our sympathy for the addict, it must be asserted that continuance of the addiction is just as agonizing for the addict, though in a different way. So first the addict wrestles with the agony and the ecstasy; and then, when the pleasures of the addictive drug are no more, he wrestles with two different kinds of agony. At no point in the proceedings is his situation merely petty or banal. In his literary reminiscences, De Quincey says of Coleridge that he sometimes thought he could abandon the habit in a week, producing what De Quincey calls "so mighty a revolution." De Quincey goes on to ask, "Is Leviathan so tamed?"

Thus hyperbole enters the language of addiction, not least in descriptions of the "agonies" of withdrawal, never to leave it again, at least not in anything likely to be read by the general public. Perhaps Coleridge was the king of hyperbole.

> O infinite in the depth of darkness, an infinite craving, an infinite capacity of pain and weakness.... O God save me—save me from myself ... driven up and down for seven dreadful Days by restless Pain, like a Leopard in a Den, yet the anguish and remorse of Mind was worse than the pain of the whole Body—O I have had a new world opened to me, in the infinity of my own Spirit!

This is the kind of self-dramatizing language in which it is impossible to tell the truth, the kind of language that someone like Princess Diana, histrionic to her finger-tips, at least when advantageous, might have used had she been born in the romantic era. (Psychobabble is perhaps its pale modern equivalent.) It is grandiose, self-pitying, exhibitionist, grotesquely self-important, and complacent in its assessment of the significance of the writer's own experience. And, precisely as one might have suspected from a passage like the above, Coleridge was indeed a terrible liar and cheat when it came to his habits of consumption. He routinely deceived his medical advisers and others who were trying to help him cut down, while swearing that he was taking no more than they allowed him. He used all kinds of subterfuges to obtain extra supplies, diverting the attention of those who were supposed to watch over him. He was as unscrupulous in this as any modern heroin addict.

One of his famous poems, "The Pains of Sleep," relates the horrors of sleep and dreams under the influence of opium (as we shall see, the part played by alcohol in laudanum consumption is often forgotten). Let us just say for now that Coleridge is not given to understatement:

> ... the fiendish Crowd
> Of Shapes and Thoughts that tortur'd me!
> Desire with loathing strangely mixt,
> On wild or hateful Objects fixt:
> Pangs of Revenge, the powerless Will,
> Still baffled, and consuming still,
> Sense of intolerable Wrong,
>
> And men whom I despis'd made strong,
> Vain-glorious threats, unmanly Vaunting,
> Bad men my boasts and fury Taunting.
> Rage, sensual Passion, mad'ning Brawl,
> And Shame, and Terror, over all!
> Deeds to be hid that were not hid,
> Which, all confus'd I might not know,
> Whether I suffer'd or I did:
> For all was Guilt, Remorse, and Woe,
> My own or others, still the same,
> Life-stifling Fear, Soul-Stifling Shame.

Coleridge was a very good poet, of course, but literal truth is not to be found in his words, especially on this subject. "The Pains of Sleep," however, might be a reasonable poetic description of delirium tremens, the withdrawal syndrome from alcohol, in which frightening visual hallucinations occur, as they do not occur in withdrawal from opiates, and indeed Coleridge is sometimes described as having hands that shook so violently that he was scarcely able to hold a glass in his hand. Shaking is a prominent symptom of withdrawal from alcohol, but not from opiates, and it is known that Coleridge drank in addition to taking laudanum. Indeed, he drank not only two pints of laudanum per day—laudanum is tincture of opium in spirits—but bibbed claret in copious quantities. The profuse sweating that he suffered, and the shaking, was much more likely to be as a result of his drinking than of his opium consumption. One way—indeed, in his time the only way—of aborting an episode of delirium tremens was to take alcohol, which perhaps explains why he felt very much better after he had had a deep draught of laudanum. It was the alcohol it contained that he imperatively needed, not the opium. As we have seen, withdrawal from alcohol is incomparably worse than that from opiates, with very real dangers. In extenuation of Coleridge, he might not have fully appreciated the different parts played by alcohol and opium in his condition.

But of course, alcohol had few romantic possibilities. It wasn't exotic, and everyone, practically, took it. To be a mere drunk was not compatible with the Romantics' thirst for world-significant angst. M.H. Abrams quotes Coleridge on the philosophic wonders of opium:

> The poet's eye in his tipsy hour
> Hath a magnifying power.
> Or rather emancipates his eyes
> Of the accidents of size.
> In unctuous cone of kindling coal,
> Or smoke from his pipe's bole,
> His eye can see
> Phantoms of sublimity.

Abrams is anxious in a footnote to make it perfectly clear that Coleridge means opium, not alcohol, when he writes of tipsiness. Almost everyone being familiar with the effects of alcohol, few would take very seriously, indeed most would laugh at, the idea that a drink or drunkenness gave poets a special insight into worlds beyond the world (though for myself, I do sometimes experience a quasi-oceanic feeling on taking my first drink after a particularly hard day dealing with, amongst others, drug addicts).

Suffice it to say that I have seen hundreds of cases both of delirium tremens and withdrawal from opiates, and Coleridge's description, in so far as it fits anything, fits the former much better than the latter. I have never witnessed an opiate addict experience frightening visual hallucinations, but I have witnessed many alcoholics (mostly men) in a state of real terror at their visual hallucinations, which often start as exceptionally vivid dreams or nightmares, imaginary beings and events that are all too real to them. Indeed, I have known such patients dive through windows of the upper stories of my hospital in order, as they supposed, to escape the monsters, or enemies, who pursued or were attacking them. (Interestingly, it has proved difficult to persuade the hospital administration that such patients should be nursed on the ground floor as a precautionary measure, suggesting a subliminal death wish, though not on the part of the patients.)

But this is not a field in which truth triumphs in the end. Rather, it is a field in which myths and inaccuracies pass down the generations, uncorrected by critical thought. Again, I give examples in the appendix.

The untruth of literary and cinematic representations of withdrawal from opiates is deeply harmful. Anyone watching or reading such misrepresentations who was without medical knowledge or experience would almost certainly come to the conclusion that no one could be expected voluntarily to go through the experience of withdrawal as depicted, at least without a vast apparatus of care. It would, indeed, be cruel to expect anyone to do so. By implication, more drug clinics are necessary to help the poor addicts avoid such traumatic experiences.

Perhaps it is not surprising that no heroin addict ever comes forward to correct the impression left by such portrayals of opiate withdrawal. Any such person would be regarded by his 'community' of fellow-addicts in much the same light as a police informer is viewed by the criminal fraternity. It serves the purposes of drug addicts to let the general public think that withdrawal entails such suffering that, in continuing their habit, addicts are actually victims in need of sympathy and medical assistance. Nor, as far as I know, has any member of the treatment profession or industry ever come forward to protest at the ridiculous exaggeration and inaccuracy of these portrayals. It would hardly serve the interests of the profession or industry to do so: the public must be misinformed if the profession or industry is to flourish. This silence reinforces the self-deception of the addicts, who both know that withdrawal is not a serious medical condition and believe that it is deadly serious at the same time. Coleridge was an early exponent of this curious doublethink: he thought he would die if he gave up opium, though at the same time he knew that he had once withdrawn from it without dying. (Of course, if it was delirium tremens from which he suffered, he might have been right, without of course knowing that he was, since he attributed all his sufferings to opium.)

There has been a continuous and unbroken literary tradition of more or less hysterical accounts of the difficulties of withdrawal. De Quincey is, of course, a famous exemplar of this school of self-exculpatory exaggeration, the phenomena of withdrawal in turn justifying the metaphor of addiction, over and over again, as slavery or enchainment.

De Quincey says with regard to withdrawal, *inter alia:*

> It will occur to you often to ask, why I did not release myself from the horrors of opium, by leaving it off, or diminishing it? ... The reader may be sure ... that I made attempts innumerable to reduce the quantity. I add, that those who witnessed the agonies of those attempts, and not myself, were the first to beg me to desist ... further reduction causes intense suffering.

And:

> The reader is aware that opium had long ceased to found its empire on spells of pleasure; it was solely by the tortures connected with the attempt to abjure it, that it kept its hold.

Note that the opium is the more active and powerful party in the transaction between it and De Quincey, and that here we see, perhaps for the first time in public, the ascription by an addict of agency to the substance which he takes. ("The beer went mad," as one of my alcoholic patients put it, or "The heroin took over," as many addicts have told me. "Not the opium-eater," says De Quincey, "but the opium, is the true hero of this tale.")

> [I]t might be sufficient to say that intolerable bodily suffering had totally disabled [me] for almost any bodily exertion.

Nor is suffering over once opium has been abjured:

> Think of me, even when four months had passed, still agitated, writhing, throbbing, palpitating, shattered; and much, perhaps, in the situation of him who has been racked [i.e., tortured on the rack].

It is difficult to think of anyone writhing, throbbing, and palpitating for four months, at least without a very severe psychiatric or neurological condition, from neither of which De Quincey suffered. What he really suffered from was Romanticism, with its inherent tendency to mistake the minor fluctuations of emotional state consequent upon the condition of being human for seismological events to be measured, or at least spoken about, on the Richter scale. Not only does he make no moral distinction between sufferings that are self-inflicted and those inflicted by others, but— a precursor of all those who so lightly and frivolously use the Holocaust as metaphor for their own suffering—he magnifies his own sufferings so as to give the impression that no one has or could ever have suffered more than he. Here is a typically trashy passage of *Suspiria de Profundis*, that, had it not been so verbose, would have been worthy of a women's magazine, describing yet another relapse into (or rather return to, since the word "relapse" implies something that happens to a person rather than something that he does) his habit and attempt to foreswear it:

> During this third prostration before the dark idol, and after some years, new and monstrous phenomena began slowly to arise ... when I could no longer conceal from myself that these dreadful symptoms were moving forward forever, by a pace steadily, solemnly, and equably increasing, I endeavoured, with some feeling of panic, for a third time to retrace my steps. But I had not reversed my motions for many weeks before I became profoundly

aware that this was impossible.... I saw through vast avenues of gloom those towering gates of ingress, which hitherto had always seemed to stand open, now at last barred against my retreat, and hung with funeral crape. The sentiment which attends the sudden revelation that *all is lost!* silently is gathered up into the heart; it is too deep for gestures or words.... I, at least, upon seeing those awful gates closed and hung with draperies of woe, as for a death already past, spoke not, nor started nor groaned.

But he did write *Suspiria de Profundis,* and quite a lot beside, and furthermore lived another fourteen years, in a state not devoid of domestic happiness. Like Coleridge, he wrote attitudinizing prose whose object was not to convey meaning but to convey an impression. And it certainly does not offer much hope to or for other addicts: "it," that is to say abstinence, is "impossible," the way of expressing it implying that the impossibility is a brute natural fact like Mount Etna or the Mariana Trench. In De Quincey's words are foreshadowed all the dishonest self-pity of subsequent addicts.

The Literary Tradition: Its Effect

Where De Quincey and Coleridge led, many others followed, almost without interruption. And repetition is a guarantee of truth, psychologically-speaking if not logically-speaking. As the Bellman puts it in "The Hunting of the Snark," "What I say three times is true." I have insisted upon this long literary tradition because I believe it to be the *fons et origo* of our mistaken ideas about addiction. Two possible objections are that, for all its error, the literary tradition to which I refer portrays addiction as a horrible condition, which no one would wish on himself; and second that it is most unlikely that many addicts have read much of it.

It is true that the tradition portrays addiction as being horrible, but it exaggerates the joys of addictive substances also, not only suggesting that they entail philosophical insight, but that there is a tragic grandeur in the very abyss between the happiness and the misery that addictive drugs give rise to, a tragic grandeur only available to great souls and not to petty natures such as yours or mine.

Moreover, there is something deeply attractive, at least to quite a lot of people, about squalor, misery, and vice. They are regarded as more authentic, and certainly more exciting, than cleanliness, happiness and virtue. We have seen that William Burroughs, the St. Louis Gnostic, was positively attracted by evil. The web site of Melvin Burgess, the author of *Junk*, a novel about heroin for twelve- to fourteen-year-olds, has a picture of him dressed in the current uniform of the slums, sitting against a wall covered in graffiti. Since he must by now have made considerable sums of money from his book (and other books), it is unlikely that he did not have the means to dress more smartly, or the bus fare to go somewhere more attractive to be photographed. His decision to present himself thus is therefore a deliberate and calculated endorsement of the world from which young drug addicts are most likely to come, and which is most likely to increase his sales. His greatest fear, or nightmare, is not to be thought hip or cool, and if to avoid that terrible fate it means that he has to glamorize evil—well, so be it.

Second, it is not necessary for people to have read certain books for them to be influential. Not everyone who speaks of Adam and Eve has read Genesis. How many people who talk of Keynesian economics have actually read Keynes? Keynes himself said that politicians are seldom doing anything but putting into practice the defunct ideas of past economists. As it happens, Coleridge thought that De Quincey's book had a Werther effect, that is to say a direct imitative effect on many young men (Werther, in Goethe's *The Sorrows of Young Werther,* committed suicide because of unrequited love, and soppy romantic young men of the time who read the novel likewise killed themselves, thinking they were doing something beautiful). But it is not necessary for the effect to have been direct for it to have been exerted: the ideas first enunciated by De Quincey and then elaborated by his followers have become part of what everyone "knows."

The narratives that addicts now tell, at least in certain circumstances, follow very closely the pattern first laid down by De Quincey. These narratives are deeply evasive, just as his was, as to how addiction started and why it continues. Do addicts seek to obtain pleasure or to avoid pain? It is now one, now the other, depending on which answer appears more advantageous at the time. The exaggeration of the pleasures and pains of opiate addiction started with him, and continues to this day: when you listen to addicts talking among themselves, they speak as if they had enjoyed the bliss of heaven, but when they speak to a doctor, they speak as if they now suffered the pains of hell. The sense of being apart from, and superior to the rest of humanity as a consequence of the experience of addiction started with De Quincey, and has continued. The preposterous inflation of the agonies of withdrawal has been accepted uncritically ever since. When it comes to drug addiction, literature has trumped—and over-trumped—pharmacology, history, and common sense.

If I am right, I have demonstrated something that has proved irritatingly difficult to demonstrate down the ages: the importance of literature. It can do a great deal of harm; whether it can do any good is, of course, another question entirely.

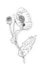

III

The Show Must Go On

*This . . . is an insanity which none but the soul's Physician
can cure. . . . The restraint which alone could efficiently
cure is that which no person can impose . . .*

—Robert Southey,
Letter to Joseph Cottle, April 1814

I argue that our current misconceptions of opiate addiction depend
upon the systematic disregard of the most obvious evidence, and
rely to a large extent upon the dishonest, exhibitionist and self-
dramatizing claptrap of the early nineteenth-century Romantics,
particularly De Quincey and Coleridge. These misconceptions,
kept alive by an almost unbroken succession of authors, some of
them medical, are not without practical consequences, for upon
them rests an entire costly and ineffectual apparatus of so-called
care. This apparatus, by disguising from the addict the real nature
of his problem, serves not only to prolong, but to spread it.
Three questions remain to be answered. The first is why a purely
literary tradition should have triumphed so completely over pharmacological and other branches of knowledge, and even over
common sense itself. The second concerns the real nature of opiate addiction itself. What are its origins and true causes? The third
concerns what practical consequences a more honest understanding of the problem would entail.

The Self-Interested and Uncritical Acceptance of Romaniticism

There is no definitive explanation for the pseudo-authority with
which Coleridge, De Quincey, et al., have been invested on this
subject. The initial acceptance of their word, when their mode of

expression was so obviously hyperbolic, and when what they wrote was internally inconsistent and self-contradictory, is no doubt partially to be explained by the Zeitgeist of their time. There was a general revolt against the cool classicism of the previous age, and sensibility triumphed over sense.

In defense of the Romantics, it might be urged that they knew less of the pharmacology of opiates than succeeding generations. For example, they were unable to distinguish between the withdrawal effects of opium and alcohol. And perhaps De Quincey really did not know that the discomforts of withdrawal (that he magnified into agonies, mere discomfort being beneath him) would not last forever: though the same cannot be said of Coleridge, who had several periods of abstinence and therefore knew perfectly well that the withdrawal period was short.

There is, however, no longer any excuse for taking them or their intellectual heirs and imitators seriously as observers of their own condition. We know, or ought to know, that they mythologized wildly, as do their followers to this day. But why is this mytholgizing treated with a respect it does not deserve, as if it were no less than the literal truth?

It serves different functions for different groups of people, of course, who have varying but compatible, indeed interdependent and synergistic, interests to defend. The originators of the myths wanted to dramatize their own lives, to raise them above the level of the mundane. For all that they had brilliant, or at least glittering gifts, Coleridge and De Quincey were utter failures by the standards they set themselves, namely to make serious and important contributions to philosophy. They probably knew at some level of their minds that such contributions were beyond their powers, but preferred to establish an external cause of their failure, as being less wounding to their pride. What better reason, or rather excuse, for their failure than "the trammels of opium." It wasn't me, says De Quincey, it was the opium:

> [the opium-taker's] intellectual apprehension of what is possible infinitely outruns his power, not of execution only, but even of the power to attempt.

In other words, I'm a genius, but unfortunately the opium—than which, as Cocteau puts it, emphasizing the passive victim status of the taker, "no mistress is more demanding" and which "carries jealousy to the point of castrating [the taker]"—got to me first and prevented me from producing the awe-inspiring, profound, and imperishable masterpieces of human thought that I should otherwise have produced. I couldn't help it; I'm a victim, and the pains of withdrawal prove it.

Banality is turned into romance and weakness into tragedy. But all is not quite lost, for as Cocteau once again puts it:

> It may happen that the smoker is a masterpiece. A masterpiece which does not discuss itself. A perfect masterpiece, because it is fugitive, without form and without judges.

Fortunate indeed! Having (possibly, only possibly) become a masterpiece by taking opiates, nothing further can seriously be demanded of the addict, and only grosser natures would demand anything so vulgar as actual work to prove it.

Of course, not all writers who have treated of opiate addiction have themselves been addicts. With very few exceptions, however, they have accepted uncritically the standard view of addiction whose essential underpinnings are the Romanticism of the early nineteenth century. (Notably, Somerset Maugham, a highly observant man not given to romantic exaggeration, described an opium den in his book of Chinese travels, *On a Chinese Screen,* as being clean, cheerful, elegant, and relaxed, quite the reverse of what the average reader must have been expecting and no doubt hoping for.) So why have most writers accepted the standard view, without so much as pause for thought?

In the first place, they are more likely to have met addicts than to have considered the question of addiction from a pharmacological, historical, or sociological perspective. Since addicts usually present themselves in the Romantic mode, as suffering terribly, as being enslaved and enchained, and since in addition they have often sunk to the bottom of the social scale, and since furthermore they are often despised by much of the surrounding society, the writers clearly consider it their duty (and, of course, their pleasure) to present the addict sympathetically, which means—for reasons I shall adumbrate—taking him at his own word and estimate. The sympathetic presentation of the opiate addict, which is to say with an uncritical attitude to the facts of the case, achieves more than one end for the non-addicted author. First it demonstrates his ability to enter imaginatively and empathically into the experience of people quite different from himself, which is an ability that all writers of fiction should have in abundance. Second it allows him to demonstrate a personal knowledge of the lower depths, which has increasingly become a requirement for an imaginative writer to be taken seriously, at least in literary circles. We do not live in an auspicious age for the likes of Jane Austen or Henry James: we want raw reality now, and raw reality is necessarily wretched. Third, it allows the author to take his distance from what he assumes are conventional moral attitudes, without realizing that the opposite of a convention is often—well, another convention. (I do not mean to imply, of course, that no challenge to conventional morality or wisdom is ever justified. It often is, and I suppose that I am doing precisely that in this book. But conventions should be challenged on the grounds of evidence, reason, and justice, not from a desire to distinguish oneself from the common herd. As Fitzjames Stephens put it, originality consists in thinking for yourself, not in thinking differently from other people.)

The non-addicted writer who accepts the standard view is in effect awarding himself the palm for thought, feeling, magnanimity, and moral philosophy.

As for the addicts themselves, it is not very difficult to see why they should accept the standard view with its pillars of Romanticism. The appeal for them is obvious. As with its originators and subsequent authors, it serves more than one function.

It suggests to them firstly that, below the surface squalor of their lives, there lies something worthwhile, perhaps even infinitely or uniquely worthwhile, depths that other people have not had the courage to plumb. They are like explorers who have travelled to remote regions, impelled by sheer curiosity and the desire to add to the sum of their own and humanity's knowledge. Necessarily, they return home slightly the worse for wear. Baudelaire tells us how worthwhile it all was:

Amazing travellers! What noble tales
Can we read in the oceanic depths of your eyes!
Show us the caskets freighted with memories,
Those marvellous jewels made out of stars and space.

We want to travel without steam or sail!
To brighten the tedium of our prison cells,
Project on to our minds, tight as sailcloth,
All your horizon-framed recollections.

Tell us: what have you seen?

(But exactly what are the marvellous jewels brought back from the drug-propelled journeys round a person's skull? *Naked Lunch*, perhaps? It is to literature what vomit is to haute cuisine.)

There is, naturally, a slight contradiction between a journey undertaken for motives of philosophical exploration, and the process of "falling in with the wrong crowd," or the other supposedly adventitious reasons addicts give for having first taken opiates. This a confusion that appears—repeatedly, as it happens—in Coleridge and De Quincey, who can never quite make up their mind as to why they first took opium. Whose life, however, is not a chapter of accidents, good and bad, fortunate and unfortunate?

The penalty paid for these daring journeys into these marvellous continents of subjectivity is, it goes almost without saying, enchainment, slavery, etc. Enchainment means that escape is impossible, and everyone knows how few successful slave revolts there have been in history. The best that an average slave can hope for is manumission, though of course manumission is entirely in the hands of others, such as the professionals in the drug clinics who proffer help. If it turns out that it is in fact beyond their powers to grant such manumission, what more can the addict do than continue in his slavery?—which is all he wanted to do in the first place.

Dramatic accounts of withdrawal are grist to the same romantic mill. An addict often finds it necessary to claim that he wants to abandon his habit. His relatives, wife, or girlfriend seeks assurances that he wants to do so as a condition of not refusing him further contact with them; various functionaries of the therapeutic agencies demand ritual assurances of attempts at reform. Meanwhile, he wants, and knows that he wants, to continue as before.

The supposed horrors of withdrawal help him to resolve this contradiction. He would do as he ought to do, and as others want him to do, but for the yawning chasm or unscalable cliff of withdrawal that lies before him. Once again, Baudelaire puts it succinctly:

> the pains [of withdrawal are] exhausting and unendurable, and deliverance was always there, within easy reach.

For the benefit of the morally obtuse, Baudelaire points the moral:

> [M]ay he among you who is without sin, either in thought or deed, be the first to throw a stone at our invalid.

Invalid: yes, the addict is an invalid, a genuinely sick person, someone who needs treatment, the terrible physical consequences of withdrawal being proof of it—the most important proof of it. Which of you, Baudelaire challenges his readers, would willingly go through such agony?

So it is hardly surprising that addicts have seized upon the standard view, with its Romantic foundations, with such alacrity. It serves their ends admirably (which is not to say that is serves their best interests). But why should doctors, who above all people are supposed to respect evidence and truth, and their sidekicks, the auxiliary drug-addiction workers such as counsellors, social workers, psychologists, nurses, etc., have accepted the whole edifice of misconceptions? Are not the muted statements of their own textbooks enough to give them pause?

Doctors are, of course, only human, however much they may sometimes try to present themselves as being above the earthly fray, or human weakness and pettiness. If you prick them do they not bleed, if you tickle them do they not laugh? And are they not prey to the same vanities and ambition for distinction as other men?

Coleridge spent the last sixteen years of his life as a paying guest and patient of the surgeon, Dr. James Gillman. The latter was a man hitherto of no very great distinction in his profession, even if he was well-enough respected, and he was of no very great scientific attainment. To have one of the great poets (and reputed thinkers) of his age as a paying guest and patient was therefore his best, perhaps his only, hope of entering the historical record. To do so, however, he had to succeed where other doctors before him had failed; success in this context meant keeping Coleridge as a patient for a long time, as long as possible. A modern drug-worker would call it "engaging Coleridge in treatment," even if his condition at the end of such treatment were not so very different from his condition at the beginning of it.

Where Dr. Gillman differed from his predecessors, apparently, was in his sympathetic, not to say gullible, acceptance of Coleridge's account of himself and his sufferings (he was also a cultivated man with literary tastes). Coleridge told him what he wanted to hear, Dr. Gillman listened and then reflected back to Coleridge what he wanted to hear. Coleridge was impressed that at last he had found a doctor who knew what he was talking about, i.e., sucking up to Coleridge.

Apart from a favorable mention in posterity, the doctor no doubt was able to indulge in a pleasing feeling of superiority to his colleagues: he had "succeeded" where they had failed. Of course, since his time, empathy such as his has reached almost epidemic proportions, and is more or less a mass phenomenon. Woe betide the doctor who fails to exhibit it, or fails to make the effort! It would be tantamount to admitting professional incompetence or malpractice, with the result that doctors who deal specifically with drug addicts now ooze empathy like a sticky secretion. And so the doctor, not to destroy the illusion, is enchained, enslaved, trammeled by his own empathy, and has to comply with the wishes of those with whom he so demonstratively empathizes. If he does not, he stands revealed as lacking empathy.

The Distortions of Ersatz Empathy and Respect

It must not be supposed, however, that the addict who is empathized with in this manner necessarily likes or respects the doctor who complies with his wishes as a result of his entrapment by his own empathy. Far from it: he laughs at the doctor's naivety, though at the same time he is perfectly willing to grow "angry," which is to say, exhibit the behavioral signs of anger, if his wishes are not complied with. William Burroughs' first book, *Junkie*, gives the game away in one of the few moments of unselfconscious frankness. (On another occasion in this book, accidentally and without realizing it, Burroughs gives the game away about something else, namely withdrawal from opiates. His symptoms on one occasion are completely alleviated by a prescription of anti-histamines, though there is not the slightest pharmacological reason why they should have relieved them. Thus even the works of confirmed equivocators, dissimulators, and self-dramatizers may provide useful evidence.) Burroughs describes a fellow-addict's visit to a doctor, whom he describes as "a writing fool" or "croaker" (the argot of the time, the early 1950s), which means a doctor willing to write prescriptions of opiates for addicts:

> Roy was giving himself a long shore leave. He located a doctor in Brooklyn who was a writing fool. This croaker would go three scripts a day for as high as thirty tablets a script.

Burroughs goes on to say:

> There are several varieties of writing croakers. Some will write only if they are convinced you are an addict, other only if they are convinced you are not. Most addicts put down a story worn smooth by years of use.

I need hardly point out that "writing fool" and "croaker" are not terms of affection or respect, nor does anything in Burroughs' narrative counteract the impression of complete contempt that they convey.

It is true that Burroughs' "writing fools" are the deadbeats of the profession, mainly willing to prescribe in return for payment. But experience shows that addicts' attitudes to doctors are usually instrumental, which is to say they use them to get whatever they can out of them in a crudely manipulative fashion. Let a doctor be as sympathetic and understanding of an addict as he likes, and let the addict respond with all the social graces at his command: if, at the end of it all, the doctor refuses what the addict wants from him, he—the addict—will turn on him like a cobra striking at its victim. He didn't come for a chat and sympathy, he came for drugs, and if he didn't get them, everything else was a waste of time. He was prepared to tolerate the doctor's intrusive entry into his private affairs if it was the price of drugs; otherwise, not.

The distorting hall of mirrors in which everyone deceives and half-deceives everyone, including himself, everyone lies and half-lies, raises expectations and then dashes them, pretends to feel what he does not feel, says what he does not think and thinks what he does not say, and yet gives no sign of the slightest awareness of any of this while being aware of it all the time, is the Romantics' legacy to the world, at least with regard to opiate addiction.

Doctor-Addicts

There is, however, another historical circumstance that reinforced doctors' willingness to see in drug addiction more than just a banal manifestation of human weakness. When, in the last quarter of the nineteenth century, the use of the hypodermic syringe and needle became widespread, doctors were the first to avail themselves of a new opportunity to addict themselves to morphine (a purified product of opium). Dr. Oscar Jennings, who was the doyen of the addiction doctors of the time, wrote this in his monograph on the subject:

> Notwithstanding the fact that one medical man out of four is a drug *habitué*, usually a morphinist, that the proportion of medical addicts to the total number of cases is in some statistics as high as ninety per cent, and that one fifth of the mortality in the profession said to be caused by morphinism, etc. etc.

This is likely to have been a gross exaggeration, but nevertheless the problem among medical men was real enough. But it could hardly be argued at the time, when medical men were striving for the utmost respectability in bourgeois society, that they were guilty en masse for anything as jejune as human weakness in the face of temptation. The profession could entertain no such simple explanation. The morphine-addicted doctor had therefore to suffer from a bona fide illness, namely morphinism, and the Romantic tradition gave credence to it. (Freud notoriously suggested cocaine as a cure for morphinism.) But the moral absolution that doctors granted themselves could scarcely be withheld from others who acted in the same way. And so there was a hardening of both lay and medical misconceptions.

Since then, as we have seen, a small but tenacious vested interest has been created. Doctors still play at being more-empathic-than-thou in their dealings with addicts, claiming to understand, and therefore to excuse, what others would only condemn: the Romantic cult of feeling, or at least the expression of feeling, still exerting its dark influence upon them.

Auxiliary Workers' Need for Addicts

The Romantic viewpoint is even more essential to that strange band of auxiliary workers who assist doctors in their efforts to "treat" addicts. In my experience, at least, they admire the addicts' rejection of bourgeois conventionality (which is still believed to be monolithic or hegemonic, as if we still lived in Ibsen's Norway, though it has long since shattered into a thousand fragments). This unconditional admiration for rebellion is itself a legacy of Romanticism, but unfortunately for the auxiliary drug workers, they do not have the courage to revolt except vicariously, through what they call their "clients." They wish to keep a foot—which is to say, a house and a salary—in the despised bourgeois world because it is so comfortable (or at least more comfortable than anything else on offer). They resolve the conflict between their incompatible desires by choosing the drug-addiction field to work in.

They try to resemble the addicts as closely as possible. They dress like them, think like them, and talk like them. They use their argot under the pretense that to do so demonstrates that they are "non-judgmental" (in fact it demonstrates that they have made a judgment—the wrong one). They are like social anthropologists who go to learn about a tribe of primitive head-hunters by means of participant observation, who claim to be agnostic on the moral character of headhunting.

It goes without saying that the auxiliary workers have a vested interest in the standard view of opiate addiction. If the Romantics were wrong, they have no job. Nothing frightens such a worker more than an addict who thinks on his own initiative and decides to give up drugs and drug workers alike. Recently on our ward in the general hospital there was a patient who had been injecting herself with heroin for about twenty years, ever since she was a teenager. She had been prescribed methadone in high doses by a drug clinic for almost as long, and continued to take it, despite continuing to inject heroin. She took a variety of other drugs as well, including cannabis, cocaine, and benzodiazepines. In the meantime, she had contracted both Hepatitis B and C, and had had several children removed from her at birth by social workers.

Altogether, then, not a therapeutic triumph. But when she told her drug counsellor, who came to visit her on the ward, that she was sick of drugs and wanted finally to reduce her dose of methadone, the counsellor grew alarmed and angry when she insisted, telling her that to cut down would be an extremely dangerous thing to do. This, after nearly two decades of prescriptions and guided navel-gazing! It could have dire consequences for her.

Dire consequences for whom? Worse than having her children taken away from her? Worse than contracting Hepatitis B and C? No: the danger was the bad example she would set if she did as she threatened. If other addicts followed suit, what future would there be for drug clinics?

At a meeting not long ago in my hospital to decide the hospital's policy on prescribing opiates to drug addicts admitted for other reasons, I raised my objections to "treatment" with methadone. "But," exclaimed one of the doctors present, a medical member of the drug addiction industry-cum-bureaucracy, "that is against the consensus"—as if we were trying to present a united political front to the world rather than thinking about what was best for people. Dressed with studious casualness, to demonstrate his distance from bourgeois conventions, he did not hesitate to appeal to convention when his interests were at stake.

A friend of mine, who worked at an institute in Scotland for the study of alcohol abuse, which is by tradition regarded as being extremely prevalent there, discovered by his research that it was no more (or less) prevalent than in the south-east of England. He presented his findings at a meeting in the institute; and at the end of his presentation, one of the staff stood up and said, "I think your research is extremely dangerous." Dangerous for the funding of the institute, that is, for it was premised on the idea that Scotland had a problem all its own. Such is the intellectual honesty often to be found in the field of addiction.

A loss of job for a drug-worker would be not only a loss of income, however important that might be. It would also be a loss of the sense of moral superiority that such people often feel with regard to those who do not "understand" drug addicts. The claim to understand what is beyond the metaphysical understanding of hoi polloi is one of the marks, as well as pleasures, of a priesthood.

Lay Sentimentality

But has not hoi polloi itself been affected—I almost said "infected"— by the standard view? Indeed it has, but usually in inverse strength and proportion to its actual contact with opiate addicts. Unless people have a vested interest in the standard view, it tends to melt away as something insubstantial on contact with reality, for example with an addicted relative.

Why is there such wide acceptance of it? For many of the reasons that non-addicted writers accept it. In addition, there is very little opposition to it: it has become an almost unassailable dogma. Moreover, the public likes victim groups on which it can expend compassion vicariously, at no real cost to itself. But in order for victim groups to be worthy of compassion, they must be entirely free of blame or responsibility for their misfortunes. It is the blamelessness of victims that confers their high moral standing. That is why the imagery of addiction as enslavement is so popular.

Besides, which of us has no bad habits that we have failed to conquer or abjure? Would we not like them to be seen in the same supposedly charitable light, not as evidence of weakness but of illness? All manner of bad habits now partake of the excul-patory rhetoric of addiction. When we say that opiate addiction is an illness that requires treatment, we prepare absolution in advance for ourselves.

And if addiction is a medical problem, then it has a medical solution. This means that disturbing non-technical questions, about the purpose of human existence, and the dark underside of our material prosperity, can be avoided. No one wants to look too closely into his own void. It is up to others to find the solution.

In sum, the standard view, created on the foundations laid by the Romantics, has been gratefully accepted as a gift by vari-ous groups—authors, addicts, doctors, and drug-addiction work-ers, and the general public—all with different axes to grind.

The True, Existential Nature of Addiction

We turn now to the second of the three questions: What is the true nature and cause of opiate addiction? We have seen that the physiological component, with which medicine as a discipline might legitimately concern itself, is small and insignificant. For once, De Quincey is quite clear. He took a dose for toothache that had become "excruciating rheumatic pains of the head and face."

> But I took it:—and in an hour, oh! heavens! . . . what an apoca-lypse of the world within me! That my pains had vanished, was now a trifle in my eyes:—this negative effect was swallowed up in the immensity of those positive effects which had opened up before me—in the abyss of divine enjoyment thus suddenly revealed. Here was a panacea . . . for all human woes: here was the secret of happiness, about which philosophers had disputed for so many ages, at once discovered: happiness might now be bought for a penny, and carried in the waistcoat pocket: portable ecstasies might be had corked up in a pint bottle: and peace of mind could be sent down in gallons by the mail coach.

Happiness at a penny a bottle! Good value indeed: who would not buy a gallon at that price? De Quincey goes on to say:

the tumult, the fever, and the strife were suspended; a respite granted from the secret burthens of the heart; a Sabbath of repose; a resting from labours. Here were the hopes which blossom in the paths of life, reconciled with the peace which is the grave . . . infinite activities, infinite repose.

And finally comes the most famous passage in the book, a dithyramb to opium:

> Oh! Just, subtle, and mighty opium! that to the hearts of poor and rich alike, for the wounds that will never heal, and for "the pangs that tempt the spirit to rebel," bringest an assuaging balm; eloquent opium! that with thy potent rhetoric stealest away the purposes of wrath; and to the guilty man, for one night givest back the hopes of his youth, and hands washed pure from blood; and to the proud man, a brief oblivion for wrongs unredress'd, and insults unavenged . . . . Thou only givest these gifts to man; and thou hast the keys of Paradise, oh, just, subtle, and mighty opium!

This is really rather better than everyday life, even for the most fortunately placed, let alone the denizens of slums.

The later nineteenth-century French medical writer on morphinism, Dr. Chambard, to whom I shall refer again, makes similar points, but in prose less heated, flamboyant, exhibitionist—and in my opinion, better. He starts out with a general reflection on man's existential situation:

> The king of the animals pays dearly for his supremacy and his power: he knows sadness, curiosity and boredom. He has also sought, at all times and in all places, a means to escape his consciousness of his own misery; he has found three such means: death, action and dream. The first requires courage; the second, energy; the third is within the reach of all, and the "poisons of the intelligence" offer the man who wishes to forget life resources that are practically inexhaustible.

And then he describes the "poisons of the intelligence," amongst which morphine is but one:

the modern slave who forgets his misery by rolling under a tavern table, the condemned man who smokes furiously while awaiting the hour of his execution, the worldly man who contemplates existence through the gilded prism of a champagne glass, the Chinese scholar whose thought floats on a blue cloud of opium, the sensual Turk for whom a spoonful of madjoum [a mixture of hashish with opium, thorn apple, and nux vomica] peoples his dreams with white houris, the disappointed man of ambition who consoles himself with morphine, the little mistress who forgets her unfaithful lover by means of the syringe, are all seeking the same end by different routes: to forget pains past, present and to come, the substitution of the dull and sad realities of life by dream or sleep.

Oh, just, subtle, and mighty Chambard, who hath penetrated so swiftly to the heart of the matter! Is it not clear that he sympathizes with the predicament of people who poison their intelligence, without thereby absolving them from their responsibility for doing so, and without accepting uncritically their views of themselves?

Man's life is a permanent disappointment to him. His state of dissatisfaction, or, at least, awareness of imperfection, is a permanent feature of his existence. But in addition to his existential anxieties—What is it all for? Is there a transcendent purpose to our sojourn in this vale of tears?—he has usually added his mite to ensure that his life contains more wretchedness than it need do. No wonder he seeks that "sweet, oblivious antidote" of which Macbeth speaks to the physician:

> Canst thou not minister to a mind diseas'd,
> Pluck from the memory a rooted sorrow,
> Raze out the written troubles of the brain,
> And with some sweet oblivious antidote
> Cleanse the stuff'd bosom of that perilous stuff
> Which weighs upon the heart?

To which the physician dryly answers:

> Therein the patient
> Must minister to himself.

While undoubtedly true, this answer has not satisfied mankind down the ages, and it still seeks instantaneous heaven on earth by means of drugs. In short, the resort to intoxicants is a permanent and ineradicable temptation that arises from human nature.

Not everyone gives in to it, however, or is equally susceptible by virtue of his situation in life. The majority of people sometimes resort to intoxicants (or, like me with alcohol, resort to them every day), without letting them interfere with their ability to function in the world. Indeed, taken in moderation, they probably increase their ability to do so. But there are some people for whom the desire for the consolation of illusion, and the illusion of consolation, is constant. Having tasted of the fruit of the tree of ignorance, they proceed to gorge themselves upon it.

We have seen how William Burroughs did not think that the world was interesting enough to engage his attention in a sustained fashion. It did not come up to the mark. In his case, this was an individual, probably congenital, quirk, for he came from a class in which such an attitude was comparatively unusual, though of course far from unprecedented. But in most western societies, there is now a class in which *tedium vitae* is very common, almost normal. This is the class from which the great majority of heroin addicts now comes, not bored semi-intellectuals like Burroughs.

The young of this class are disaffected, and have good reason to be so. They are for the most part poor, though not of course in the absolute sense. On the contrary, they are healthier, better fed, dressed, and sheltered than the great majority of the world's population, past and present, and dispose of appurtenances whose sophistication would have astonished our forefathers. But they are poor in the context of their own societies (which is what counts psychologically) and they are so badly educated (this time in the absolute sense) that any historical or geographical comparison, by means of which they might put their poverty in some kind of perspective, is completely beyond them.

They have no interests, intellectual or cultural. The consolations of religion are closed to them. As for their family lives, loosely so-called, they are usually of an utterly chaotic nature, a quicksand of step-parents, step- and half-siblings, and quite without an orderly succession of generations. Their sexual relationships are a kaleidoscope of ephemeral couplings, often with abandoned offspring as a result, motivated by an immediate need for sexual release and often complicated by primitive egotistical possessiveness leading to violence and conflict. Their emotional life is intense but shallow, and their interactions with others governed by power rather than any kind of principle. Life is a matter of doing what you can get away with.

Their economic prospects are poor. They are unskilled in countries in which the demand for unskilled labour is limited. If they live in countries in which social security payments are without limit of time, work is hardly worthwhile for them: they are only marginally better off with it than without it, and much less free to dispose of their time. Any work that they do will be repetitive and dull; and while a man might once have derived satisfaction from performing a menial task well, from leading a life of modest usefulness to others, this is not an age in which such humility is very common.

In large part, this is because people live to a quite unprecedented degree in the virtual world of so-called popular culture. From the very earliest age, their lives are saturated with images of celebrities, whose attainments are often modest but who have been whisked by good fortune into a world of immense and glamorous luxury. The comparison with their own surroundings, squalid if not poor in the literal sense, is not only stark but painful, and is experienced as an open wound into which salt is continually rubbed. It is also experienced as an injustice, for why should people with tastes and accomplishments not so very different from their own lead a life of fairy-tale abundance? The injustice of which they feel themselves to be the victim reduces any lingering inhibitions against causing harm to society, which means in practice individual members of society. Crime ceases to be crime, but is rather restitution or justified revenge. And the fact that the abundance they so desire is itself empty and leads to dissatisfaction and boredom entirely escapes them.

The end result is that, while profoundly dissatisfied with their present lot, they do not have ambitions towards which they might actually work in a constructive fashion, but daydreams, in which everything is solved at once in a magical way, daydreams from which the emergence into reality is always painful. Any aid to the perpetuation of the state of daydreaming (or reverie, as Coleridge and De Quincey call it) is therefore greatly appreciated.

Other Rewards of Heroin Addiction

This is not the only compensation that life as a heroin addict gives to the susceptible, however. Quite apart from the prolongation of the state of daydreaming, and the satisfaction of doing what a despised society forbids them from doing (the vices of my enemy being my virtues), the life of the drug addict is actually quite busy and purposeful. It entails the existence of a network, if not of friends exactly, at least of similarly placed acquaintances. It creates a sense of urgency every day, for the addicts must (or, rather, feels he must) find his supplies, and it imposes a structure to the day and even a discipline. And just when the routine becomes dull, a crisis supervenes: a police raid, for example, or a turf war between suppliers. The fact is that the opiate addict enters a world of espionage and counter-espionage that lends an excitement to his sordid and petty existence, and that is in marked contrast to the artificial tranquillity brought about by the drug itself. Life is less boring with heroin than without it.

The temptation to take opiates, and to continue to take them, therefore arises from two main sources: first, man's eternal existential anxieties, to which there is no wholly satisfactory solution, at least for those who are not unselfconsciously religious; and second, the particular predicament in which people find themselves. Modern societies have created, or at least resulted in, a substantial class of persons peculiarly susceptible to what De Quincey calls "the pleasures of opium."

A distinguished American philosopher, Herbert Fingarette, wrote a book on the philosophical analysis of the concept of alcoholism as a disease. Not coincidentally, he had previously written a book on the philosophical analysis of the phenomenon of self-deception, which is easier to name than to understand. What Fingarette said of alcoholism can be applied with equal force to opiate addiction:

> Each of us has developed a particular way of life. . . . For example, I am a university professor and devote a good portion of my time to teaching, talking to students, reading, and writing . . . just as my professorial activities affect and color much of the rest of my life, so too do my other central activities color my professional conduct. . . . To say that heavy drinking is a *central activity* for someone is to say that it is an activity of the same order for the person as my vocation is for me. . . . [H]eavy drinking becomes a central activity in the drinker's life, it shapes his or her daily schedule, friendships, domestic life, and occupational choices. Heavy drinkers tend to organize their lives to minimize contact with people who frown on drinking or condemn excessive drinking.

It should be clear by now that the causes of opiate addiction, and the reasons why it is maintained, have nothing to do with medicine as a discipline. The addict has a problem, but it is not a medical one: he does not know how to live. And on this subject the doctor has nothing, qua doctor, to offer. What he ought not do, however, is to mislead the addict, or allow the addict to mislead him, into thinking that the problem is medical and requires, or is susceptible to, a medical solution.

The Inhumanity of Treatment

Contrary to our current pieties, therefore, which give those who subscribe to them a comfortable warm glow of generosity of spirit, but which are actually dehumanizing because they reduce addicts to the status of mere physiological specimens or preparations in a laboratory, addiction is a moral weakness par excellence. Moreover, addicts tend to be bad people (if bad people are those who consistently behave badly). They usually impose costs, often very severe costs, on other people without giving anything in return. Their lives are usually selfish and self-centered. Susceptibility arising from their pre-addiction circumstances is at best a mitigation, not a complete excuse. This is not to say that they are necessarily the worst people who exist, or that they are irredeemably bad (it is one of the theses of this book, after all, that they can, and often do, redeem themselves): but bad they are so long as they maintain themselves in their addiction. Addicts should therefore be stigmatized far more than they are. It is perfectly just that they should be and it could be beneficial as well, in the absence of medical "treatment."

What Is To Be Done?

We come now to the third and final question. Having argued that our current misconceptions of opiate addiction have their origins in evasive Romantic persiflage, which in turn has given rise to a pseudo-therapeutic bureaucracy that actively maintains people in their addiction and serves to spread it as a social phenomenon, I now turn to the question of what should be done. Should everything remain the same, or should there be a radical change? Should we start anew?

The question with regard to opiates that people always ask, as if a yes or a no exhausted every possibility, is whether opiates should be legalized.

The advocates of legalization seldom spell out the precise details of the proposal. Do they mean that heroin should be available on every street corner for everyone who wishes to buy it? Do they mean that the state should establish a monopoly on sales, and raise taxes thereby, or that there should be free competition between suppliers? Do they mean that heroin should be available to all, without age restrictions? Do they mean that doctors should be able to prescribe it, and if so, to anyone who asks for it or only to those who are already addicted? Or do they mean that everything should proceed on the same basis as at present, except that the law should take no cognizance of it? Legalization is not a straightforward matter.

But whatever may be meant by it, two considerations are urged in its favor. The first is that the state has no right to interfere in the private activities of its citizens, unless they harm others. The second is that most of the harmful consequences of heroin addiction arise from the illegality of heroin supply, rather than from addiction itself, and that therefore benefits—particularly a reduction in drug-related crime—would result from legalization.

Neither of these arguments is convincing. The first is an instance of the desire that there should be a simple universal principle by which all important questions may be answered. The principle in question here is the famous one enunciated in John Stuart Mill's *On Liberty:*

> The only purpose for which power may be rightfully exercised over any member of a civilized community, against his will, is to prevent harm to others. His own good, either physical or moral, is not sufficient warrant.

But no man, least of all a drug addict, is an island; we all live in society with other men. It is hard to discover activities that affect only the person who undertakes them. And while it is certainly possible for opiate addicts to lead otherwise normal lives, the fact is (and is likely to remain) that the great majority of them do not. As I have already said, they impose costs on others, often very heavy ones.

We do not find it strange or objectionable that the state, or some other public power, places restrictions on the sale and consumption of alcohol, by limits on when, where, and in what circumstances it may be sold and consumed. Indeed, we would probably find it strange if there were no such restrictions. And since the overall consumption of alcohol is price-sensitive, governments can and do encourage or discourage consumption by taxation policy. (I once worked as a doctor to the workers on a road-building project in Africa. For reasons too complex now to go into, alcohol was virtually free of charge and given *ad libitum* to the contingent of British workers on the project. I discovered that in these circumstances, about a fifth of British construction workers will regularly go to bed so drunk that they urinate in their sleep. Most of them had never drunk so heavily before.)

Few people believe that control over the sale and consumption of alcohol should be abandoned altogether, leaving it up to the law to prosecute drunken offenses only when they occur. And if the state has the right to interfere in the free market for alcohol to such an extent, it must have the right to ban its consumption altogether—though whether it would be wise to do so is another question entirely. Most people would regard such a ban to be both unwise and oppressive (oppression can result from the exercise of rights as well as from their denial). Prohibition in America did, in fact, have some benefits, such as an eventual reduction in the prevalence of alcoholic liver disease; as for the crime wave it is said to have occasioned, it is notable that the murder rate in the United States fell more in the decade before Prohibition than in the decade after it. The murder rate during Prohibition did not rise until some years into it. In other words, the relation between Prohibition and criminality was less straightforward than is suggested by the simple stimulus-response model. This should not alarm drinkers unduly, however, for there are good arguments against Prohibition. Mill's principle, however, is not among them.

If the philosophical argument against outlawing the supply of heroin fails, there might still be good prudential reasons against it. After all, wisdom and good governance require more than the consistent application of abstract principles. If the criminality associated with drug-taking were caused by the legal prohibition of supply, it might be advisable to change the law.

An association, such as that between heroin addiction and crime, is not proof of causation, however. It might be fortuitous, or dependent on a third variable, or the causative relationship might be opposite to the one first thought of. We have already seen that it is more plausible to ascribe heroin consumption to cultural antinomianism ("transgressive" is a term of praise nowadays in art criticism) or to a pre-existent propensity to criminality than the other way round. If this is the case, then legalizing the supply of heroin might not bring about the hoped-for reduction in crime.

While the average heroin-addicted criminal confines himself largely to petty crime, or crime against the owners of property, there is a group of people associated with heroin addiction who commit more serious crimes. I refer, of course, to the drug dealers. There are very few serious crimes, up to and including kidnap, torture, and murder, that they do not commit. Almost by definition, if the supply of heroin were legalized, their heroin-related criminality would be reduced.

This does not mean, however, they would cease to be criminals. Having met a fair number of drug-dealers in my time, I find it not altogether easy to believe that, if the heroin supply were legalized, they would beat their needles into ploughshares. On the contrary: they would feel obliged to turn their attention elsewhere. So long as the supply of heroin is illegal, their criminality (at least it its most violent manifestations) is directed mainly at members of what one might call the drug-dealing community, and at addicts who fail to meet their obligations. If responsibility for the supply of heroin were taken from them, they might turn their violence elsewhere. And while the death of a drug-dealer might be a tragedy for his mother who loved him, it is not really tragic for the rest of society, even if it feels obliged to weep crocodile tears over his timely demise.

All the violence inflicted by drug-dealers whose results I have witnessed in my hospital has been on other people associated in some way with the trade. Legalization might result in some of the violence spreading outwards—towards you and me, in fact.

But so long as there were some restriction on the sale of heroin (to minors under the age of eighteen, for example), a black market, with all its allegedly attendant evils, would survive. Yet other proposals, for example that doctors should prescribe heroin, but only to the already addicted, would have no effect upon the black market.

In effect, the legalizer's argument is tantamount to saying that the cause of crime is the existence of laws, and that without private households, for example, there would be no burglary.

There are two respects in which the legalizers might be right. First, a legalized supply would probably be very much purer, so that addicts would be enabled to judge their doses accurately and avoid the dangerous consequences of the changing purity of the street supply, which results in quite a number of deaths. This is to assume, of course, that making heroin addiction safe is a desirable end.

Second, if it is true that the illegality surrounding heroin addiction is one of its attractions for slum dwellers and intellectual antinomians, legalization would reduce its attractiveness. On the other hand, its illegality probably acts as a deterrent for more timid souls. If anything that reduces the costs, both financial and legal, of a psychoactive substance increases its overall consumption, and if it is desirable that as few people as possible in a society should take it, then it would be imprudent to do anything to change the legal status of the heroin supply.

On balance, therefore, I think that the arguments against legalization, however formulated, are stronger than those in favor.

Far more important in the long run than the question of legalization, however, is our attitude towards addiction. Human beings react to the predicaments in which they find (and put) themselves according to their ideas, beliefs, and values. These, though changeable, are often inherited, even though it is not known exactly from what or from whom.

On no subject has the baleful influence of the past been so strong as that of opiate addiction. Almost everything everyone knows about it is wrong, and obviously wrong. The errors are derived ultimately from the self-serving, self-dramatizing, and evasive and dishonest accounts of De Quincey and Coleridge. It is time we escaped from their shadow, nearly two centuries long.

As a first step to doing so, I would suggest the closure of all clinics claiming to treat drug addicts, the modern bureaucratic institutionalization of Romantic ideas. This would put an end to the harmful pretense that addicts are ill and in need of treatment. In the former Soviet Union, there was a saying of the workers that "We pretend to work, and they pretend to pay us." Drug addicts could say something similar to capture the reality of the current system: "We pretend to be ill, and they pretend to cure us." Henceforth, instead, doctors should treat addicts only for the serious physical complications of drug addiction: abscesses, viral infections and the like.

Addicts would then have to face the truth. Whatever their background, they are as responsible for their actions as anyone else. The truth will not necessarily set them free, but neither will it enchain them in "mind-forg'd manacles."

APPENDIX

In this Appendix, I give some examples—not exhaustive, of course, for an exhaustive catalogue would turn what is intended to be a brief essay into a weighty tome, but demonstrative of my point— of the literary tradition that has so powerfully affected popular and medical conceptions of opiate addiction, to the great detriment of truth. The literary tradition encompasses both original work and commentary upon it.

Wisdom

At the end of the nineteenth century and the beginning of the twentieth century, there was a literary fashion, especially in France, for the smoking of opium, both as an aid to philosophical insight and as a mark of membership of a bohemia morally and aesthetically superior to the stuffy world of the bourgeoisie. The ground had, of course, been prepared by Baudelaire, whose *Paradis artificiels* was in large part a loose translation and adaptation of De Quincey.

Even where the supposed insights gained are uncomfortable or frightening, they give to the man who has them an air of superiority, or at least of knowingness. Here, for example, is Jules Boissière, a colonial official in Vietnam, and himself a smoker of opium, who wrote a book of short stories in the tradition of the Decadents called *Fumeurs d'opium* (Opium Smokers). The narrator and protagonist is a man who is searching in the densely forested hills of Vietnam for ancient gold mines protected by the curse of a former king of Annam. Opium has opened his eyes to realities that he had never previously suspected:

[E]ver since I smoked opium in the forest . . . I have been afraid to die, because of what might come after. I understand so many things whose existence I never even suspected, in the blessed days of ignorant certainty and joy! [i.e. before he smoked opium]

Here the smoking of opium plays the part in Boissière's mind that the dictation of the Koran to Mohammed plays in the mind of Moslems: it put an end to the era of ignorance.

Opium has made me so clearsighted!—sometimes I pride myself on it, because I know so much more than before; but more often I suffer for it, because I have lost tranquillity of soul.

Perhaps, in this landscape where vegetation reigns, proud and absolute sovereign;—where man is of so little account, almost hardly tolerated, where he can remain only if he accepts that he will die young, as a result of the deadly miasma of the vegetation,—perhaps he survives at all only because of those mysterious influences, of which our dark Middle Ages were so aware, and because of the phantoms, driven out of the inhabited world, fled here to reign over the twilight souls of poor folk.

But how did this thought creep into my mind, I who was so confident in my materialism? Ah! It was because I smoked opium and I felt growing in me a sense that I previously lacked, that could not have developed in skeptical Europe.

I smoked more and more, to forget the fever, and to forget the phantoms. But if they had been nothing but the vain creations of my weakened brain, opium would have chased them away, no doubt, just as it had made so many ephemeral daydreams, prejudices, regrets, and senseless scruples disappear. . . . No, opium confirmed, more than ever, the existence of these phantoms, because it kills error and unmasks the truth.

In other words, the smoking of opium revealed to the narrator a world not visible to non-smokers. While he may not have been any the happier for it, he was in possession of arcane knowledge that only opium could have revealed: and what opium reveals must be true. It surely follows that, if you want to be wise in the same way, you must resort to opium.

Another French writer of the decadent school, Claude

Farrère—who has a street named after him in Istanbul, and after a character in one of whose novels the Guerlain perfume Mitsuoko is named, and who was talking to the French president Paul Doumer when he was assassinated in 1932—wrote a book of short stories called *Fumée d'opium* (published in English in 1929 as *Black Opium*). In the introduction to this volume, Pierre Louÿs, himself a poet of the soft-porn school, wrote:

> One evening, in the company of a few friends, I chanced to be at the home of a certain master-writer, when I noticed, in the middle of a table, a tall pile of manuscripts. . . .
>
> "Does that interest you?" inquired my host. "Do not ask me whose it is, for I know nothing about the author myself. A newspaper recently started a short-story contest; and a dozen judges, among whom I have the honor to be one, are charged with the task of awarding the prizes. And how many contestants do you think there are? Six thousand. Yes, six thousand manuscripts to read, accompanied by as many small envelopes, each bearing the author's emblem on the the first page . . ."

Louÿs picked up Claude Farrère's entry:

> The envelope was closed with a large bees-wax seal, along with an inscription in foreign characters, which I was unable to read. As for the prescribed author's emblem, it was as follows:
>
> LIFE: DREAM
OPIUM: REALITY

In the stories themselves, we once again hear of the philosophical properties of opium. In "The Wisdom of the Emperor," for example, a stranger offers the Emperor of China, Hoang-Ti, a pipe of opium, a drug previously unknown to him, and, finding it good, he allows it to spread among the populace:

> The opium escapes from the pipes in large puffs, wrapping the whole populace in its sublime intoxication. Under their widened foreheads, thought dwells, magnified each day by the clairvoyant drug.
>
> Beyond the city, beyond the province, and all the way to the snowy frontiers which bound the Midland Empire, the opium spreads over cities and countryside. And behold, everywhere, there

comes with it peace, tolerance, philosophy. Behold the coming of wisdom and happiness.

The Empire is founded, the Empire prospers. The triumphant people enjoy their effortless victory. And the opium teaches them mildness of repose, the joy of the gentle lassitude that languishes in the depths of layouts, under the light-winged flight of dreams, floating in the black smoke overhead. The philosophic opium tempers barbarian rudeness, renders tractable disproportioned energies, and civilizes and refines brutal impulses that are all too powerful and all too prolific.

This is pure De Quincey a century later. But it has the merit of encapsulating in two words one of the great attractions of opiates: "effortless victory." Is there anybody, really, who does not at least sometimes dream of the annihilation by pill or by inhalation of magic smoke or by some sudden, effortless coup (a win on the lottery, for example) of all the frustrations and miseries of existence?

In the story that follows, the pirate king Hong-Kop has "freed [himself] from the despised domination of Hoang-Ti." (So much for the spirit of universal benevolence and philosophic happiness brought about the opium fumes wafting over the empire.)

Deeply, Hong-Kop breathes in a divine whiff, and his eyes fill with superhuman thoughts...

How easy to achieve deep significance in one's thoughts: just breathe in!

Jean Cocteau smoked opium most of his adult life (that is, if he was ever fully adult), and wrote a book about giving up, though in the event not for good or even for very long. *Opium, the Diary of an Addict,* was published in France in 1931 and in America in 1933. Needless to say, smoking opium wasn't merely a self-indulgent habit for Cocteau: it did philosophical wonders for him too. His sense of his own superiority oozes from every line, though in most other respects the book is deeply insincere, with its sub-Wildean epigrams such as "I should greatly like to be lacking in manners. A lack of manners is the mark of the hero." On the contrary, it is the mark of the boor. With regard to opium:

The deadly boredom of the smoker who is cured. Everything that we do in life, including love, is done in an express train traveling towards death. To smoke opium is to leave the train while in motion; it is to be interested in something other than life and death.

The addict who no longer takes drugs finds life boring; and the fault, of course, is life's. But the addict penetrates deeper than the limits of our existence.

The addict is also a sensitive soul:

> To take opium ... is to escape in the spiritual domain from stupid worries which have nothing to do with discomfort in the physical domain.

Not that this is not just escapism, that is to say, escape from something unpleasant: it is escape towards something deeply significant and worthwhile in itself. And society—that is to say, those members of it not brave or intelligent enough to take opium—is envious:

> Nothing is less impure than that masterpiece: the opium smoker. Nothing is more natural than that society should demand a share, condemning it as invisible beauty, without a trace of prostitution.

And:

> Opium induces fits of wisdom.

And again:

> Naturally opium remains unique and its well-being superior to that of health. To it I owe my perfect hours.

The wisdom that opium conferred upon Cocteau did not, of course, include that of judging the Nazis, with whom he quite clearly sympathized, aright: but, of course, so small a thing as the Nazi attempt at world domination was but an epiphenomenon compared with the true and much more significant drama contained within Jean Cocteau's skull, in his opium-perfected brain.

Cocteau liked to deceive himself that there was something more refined and philosophical about opium than about other opiates, on the egotistically snobbish grounds that anything that he did was certain to be more refined than anything that others did, such as inject themselves with morphine or heroin. But in fact his habit (and that of the other writers about opiates from the standpoint of personal experience, that is to say, rationalization and self-justification) was in essence no different from anyone else's. A sense of superiority never lies very far below the surface of those who take opiates and seek to justify themselves to themselves and others.

Anna Kavan, the British writer who was a follower of Kafka and, later in life, a writer of dystopian science fiction, injected heroin for most of her adult life. Shortly after she addicted herself to the drug in 1926, aged 26, she wrote this in her diary:

> Real life is a hateful and tiresome dream ... yet how happy I might be with just a little happiness. I possess in the highest degree the art of making a little go a long way, and I am not affected by what affects other people. ...
>
> I realise completely the hopeless nature of my character. And yet, I still have a certain conceit; I still feel superior to the majority. This is curious. Perhaps I feel superior merely because I understand and analyse myself more than other people. ...

In a later story with a heroin addict for a narrator, she makes it clear that the heroin addict is, at least, superior to the cigarette smoker and the drinker:

> I think smoking and drinking are vices, disgusting habits, they're so offensive to everybody. The smell of stale smoke in our house is revolting, it clings to the curtains, the bedclothes, no matter how often they're washed. Smoke hangs inside the lampshades, turns the ceilings yellow. Then, when he drinks too much, he gets quarrelsome and aggressive, embarrasses people by stumbling about and making stupid remarks. What I do never affects anyone else. I don't behave in an embarrassing way. And a clean white powder is not repulsive; it looks pure, it glitters, the pure white crystals sparkle like snow.

In *The Connection*, a play about the lives of heroin addicts by the American playwright Jack Gelber, which was first staged in 1959, one of the addicts, an intellectual called Solly, says:

> You are fed up with everything for the moment. And like the rest of us you are a little hungry for a little hope. So you wait and worry. A fix of hope. A fix to forget. A fix to remember, to be sad, to be happy, to be, to be. ... Gallant white powder.

To be, to be: to exist in a realm of pure and unadulterated being, shorn of accidentals, without any of the contingent irritations of the petty world about us, such as utility bills and this week's shopping to be done. The heroin addict's search is something almost religious and charged with philosophical significance, therefore, a little like the saddhu's in India.

The introduction to the published version of the play was written by Kenneth Tynan, a prominent and extremely influential theater critic of the time, who was also the kind of man who could not see a taboo without trying to break it, as a personal challenge to his ego (he was the first man to utter a certain expletive on British television). In his introduction to the play, Tynan says:

> If the aim of life is pleasure, why is it more desirable to achieve it by injecting dollars into the bank account than by injecting dope into the bloodstream? If, on the other hand, the aim is spiritual enlightenment, how can we be sure that the insights provided by heroin ... are less reliable than those supplied by religious mysticism?

Now even if the aim of life were pleasure, it is surely possible to think of pleasures beyond the accumulation of money for its own sake and the psychological state brought about by the injection of heroin: this is a false, and grossly dishonest, dichotomy, and therefore makes no moral point. As for the spiritual insights "supplied" by heroin, Tynan's words assume that they exist, which is surely something that needs to be proved. What exactly are they? What immense insights does humanity owe to the millions of people who have intoxicated themselves with opiates? ("The banana is great, but the banana skin is greater"?) It might be argued, of course, that such insights are available only to the people who have them, the nature of spiritual insights being that they are ineffable and therefore incommunicable. This, however, could be urged in defense of any activity whatsoever: no matter how depraved or vicious, any practice could be claimed by its practitioners to result in some kind of personal enlightenment.

The Scottish novelist of the Beat generation Alexander Trocchi, who had a degree in philosophy, and who was a heroin addict throughout his adult life, which he spent largely in America, wrote a novel called *Cain's Book,* published in 1960. Very early on, the protagonist, a heroin addict, has sophisticated mental experiences that go to the very heart of being:

> The mind under heroin evades perception as it does ordinarily; one is aware only of its contents. But that whole way of posing the question, of dividing the mind from what it's aware of, is fruitless . . . . it is that the perceiving turns inward . . . . the blood is aware of itself, a slow phosphorescence in all the fabric of flesh and nerve and bone; it is that the organism has a sense of being intact and unbrittle, and above all, *inviolable.*

And again, a few lines later:

> I don't seriously occupy myself with the question [of the past or the future] in the "here-and-now," lying on my bunk and, under the influence of heroin, inviolable. That is one of the virtues of the drug, that it empties such questions of all anguish, transports them to another region, a painless theoretical region, a play region, surprising, fertile and unmoral. One is no longer grotesquely involved in the becoming. One simply is.

Trocchi's training as a philosopher shows, because he is an adept sophist:

> . . . the illusory sense of adequacy induced in a man by the drug. Illusory? Can a . . . "datum" be false? Inadequate? In relation to what? The facts? What facts? Marxian facts? Freudian facts? Mendelian facts? More and more I found it necessary to suspend such facts, to exist simply in abeyance, to give up (if you will), and come naked to apprehension.

So if a man believes he has achieved wisdom though the consumption of opiates, he has achieved wisdom, because no datum of experience can be false.

The Supposed Agonies of Withdrawal

It is perhaps here that literature and quasi-literary productions, such as films, are at their most egregiously inaccurate, and myths continue to be peddled, quite undisturbed by critical thought or contact with reality.

In cinematic representations of heroin withdrawal, for example, Coleridge's "The Pains of Sleep" is more or less taken as a script or template to be followed: for example in *The Man with the Golden Arm*, or more recently in the British film *Trainspotting*. In the latter, an addict who wishes to withdraw from heroin has himself locked in a room for a few days and there undergoes all the horrors of delirium tremens, with frightening visual illusions and hallucinations, together with the most terrible shakes and sweats. He has to be locked in the room, otherwise he would try to escape from them, so terrible are they, or so confused would he be. As a cinematic representation of delirium tremens it would do perfectly well; but as a representation of withdrawal from opiates, it is grotesque.

Furthermore, such misrepresentations and untruth are deeply harmful. Anyone watching a film such as *Trainspotting* who was without medical knowledge or experience, as many millions who did watch it must have been, would almost certainly have come to the conclusion that no one could be expected voluntarily to go through the experience of withdrawal as depicted, at least without a vast apparatus of medical care. It would, indeed, be cruel to expect anyone to do so. By implication, more drug clinics are necessary to help the poor addicts avoid such traumatic experiences.

The film *Trainspotting* is far from an isolated example of gross misrepresentation. Only five days before I wrote this, an episode of a British soap opera about a hospital emergency room was broadcast that portrayed a young heroin addict who wished to withdraw from heroin being brought to hospital by his parents. At first the doctors and nurses took the "cruel" view that he should be prescribed nothing; clearly, they were monsters of callousness, that is to say they were "judgmental." But they were proved wrong, because the young man then had the most terrible symptoms of withdrawal: agonizing pains, culminating in a full-blown epileptic fit. Again, the portrayal was of Coleridge's "The Pains of Sleep," and the lesson of the episode was clear:

that withdrawal is so terrible that it needs medical attention and explains why so many addicts persist in their self-destructive habit. Thus that great organ of supposed independence and objectivity, the BBC, which broadcasts the soap opera, and which is a state-run organization, perpetuates a myth that had its origins in the self-pitying vaporings of the Romantics.

The only skepticism, to my knowledge, exhibited by a famous writer with regard to opiate addiction was that of Somerset Maugham — himself a doctor, of course, though never a practicing one — who, in his marvellous book *On a Chinese Screen,* depicted an opium den in China as a clean, cheerful, and convivial place, where the Chinese congregated to have a pipe as the English, before they gave themselves over to utter brutishness, used to enjoy a convivial drink in a cozy pub.

Where De Quincey led in his exaggerations, many others have followed. He started a fashion that was followed very soon afterwards and even now has not been superseded. In 1868, for example, a man called Horace Day published anonymously a book in New York entitled *The Opium Habit, with Suggestions as to the Remedy.* This book is the origin of the idea that the Civil War was the cause of a vast epidemic of opiate addiction in the United States, as a result of the very large number of troops who received opiates for both wounds and dysenteric diseases. This is an implausible hypothesis because, as we have seen, medical use rarely leads to lasting addiction.

The first part of the book is entitled "A Successful Attempt to Abandon Opium," and is an opium memoir by the author himself. It contains a detailed account of his withdrawal from opium undertaken over several weeks. The sufferings he describes make those of Coleridge and De Quincey seem like mild inconveniences at worst.

> Matters now began to look a good deal more serious. . . . A strange compression of the stomach, sharp pains like the stab of a knife beneath the shoulder-blades, perpetual restlessness, an apparent prolongation of time . . . an incapacity of fixing the attention upon any subject whatever, wandering pains over the whole body, the jaw, whenever moved, making a loud noise, constant irritability of mind and increased sensibility to cold, with alternations of hot

flushes.... From this stage commenced the really intolerable part of the experience of an opium-eater retiring from service.... From the point I had now reached until opium was wholly abandoned, that is for a month or more, my condition may be described by the single phrase, intolerable and almost unalleviated wretchedness. Not for a waking moment during this time was the body free from acute pain; even in sleep, if it may be called sleep which much of it was little else than a state of diminished consciousness, the sense of suffering underwent little remission.... The first tears extorted by pain since childhood were forced out by some glandular weakness. Restlessness, both of body and mind, had become extreme, and was accompanied with a hideous and almost maniacal irritability.... At this time the sense of physical exhaustion had become so great that it required an effort to perform the most common act. The business of dressing was a serious tax upon the energies. To put on a coat or draw on a boot, was no light labor, and was succeeded by a feeling of prostration as required considerable time to recover from it ... the aggravation of the pain previously endured was marked. The feeling of bodily and mental wretchedness was perpetual, while the tedium of life and occasional vague wish that it might somehow come to an end were not infrequent.... The entire mental energies seemed to be exhausted in one consideration—how not to give in to the tumult of pain from which I was suffering.... The opium suffering was so great that any minor want was almost inappreciable ... the agony of pain was inexpressibly dreadful ... sleep for any duration ... was an impossibility. The sense of exhausting pain was unremitted day and night.... A perpetual stretching of the joints followed, as though the body had been upon the rack, while acute pains shot through the limbs.... During one of the last days of this protracted storm my old nervous difficulty returned in redoubled strength. Commencing in the shoulder, with its hot needles it crept over the neck and speedily spread its myriad fingers of fire over the nerves that gird the ear, now drawing their burning threads and now vibrating the tense agony of these filaments of sensation. By a leap it next mastered the nerves that surround the eye, driving its forked lightning through each delicate avenue into the brain itself, and confusing and confounding every power of thought and of will.... It was at night, however, that the suffering ... became almost unendurable ... when darkness fell ... nothing remained except a patient endurance with which to combat the strange torment.... The monotonous sound of the ticking clock often became unendurable.... At times it seemed to articulate sounds. "Ret-ri-bu-tion" I recollect as being a not uncommon burden of its song. As the racked body, and the mind, possibly beginning to be diseased, became intolerant of the odious sound, the motion of the clock was sometimes stopped, but the silence which succeeded was even worse to the disordered imagination than the voices which had preceded it. With the eyes closed in harmony with the deadly stillness, all created nature seemed annihilated, except my single, suffering self, lying in the midst of a boundless void.

Compared with this, the House of Usher was but a pleasant health resort. It comes as rather a shock, therefore, to learn a little later in the narrative that after a month of such agony:

the appearance of health and vigor had astonishingly increased. I had gained more than twenty pounds in weight.... I was repeatedly congratulated upon my healthy, vigorous condition. Few men in the entire city bore about them more of the appearance of perfect health.

Appearances are deceptive, however, for nine years later, he still suffered the following withdrawal symptoms:

1. Pressure upon the muscles of the limbs and in extremities, sometimes as of electricity apparently accumulated there under a strong mechanical force
2. A disorder condition of the liver
3. A sensitive condition of the stomach
4. Acute shooting pains, confined to no one part of the body
5. An unnatural sensitiveness to cold
6. Frequent cold perspirations in parts of the body
7. A tendency to impatience and irritability of temper, with paroxysms of excitement wholly foreign to the natural disposition
8. Deficiency and irregularity of sleep
9. Occasional prostration of strength
10. Inaptitude for steady exertion

Let us progress a few years to *Doctor Judas: A Portrayal of the Opium Habit*, published in 1895. The author, William Rosser Cobbe, was himself an addict; his book went through at least three printings, and my copy was once owned by Amos Jay Cummings who was, for much of the last part of the nineteenth century, a member of the House of Representatives and was once Chairman of the House Committee on Naval Affairs. This suggests that Cobbe's book must have reached influential people. It fully participated in the tradition of exalted exaggeration inaugurated by De Quincey.

Cobbe appears to have believed that opium (by which he meant all opiate drugs, including injectable morphine, which he also took) had plans and interests of its own, like a foreign power. In the preface to his book, he says:

> Could the victim of the insatiate drug but feel that the infliction was part of the divine harmony, he might learn to a ministration, the justice of which is to him past cognition.

And then:

> The first work of the Judas drug is to double-lock the prison door of the will, so that successful struggle against the demoniac possession is impossible.

Cobbe uses the metaphor of slavery as if it were literally true. The first words of the book proper are:

> Inexorable duty, and that alone, has urged the writer to the painful task of recording the terrible story of a nine years' slavery to opium.

Let no one accuse Cobbe of underestimating the suffering caused by opiates:

> While offering ... high testimony to the beneficent uses of opium [i.e., as an analgesic] there flashes the reflection, considering the incalculable harm which has been and is being done though its agency, does the good compensate for its harm? When the nine drear and despairing years of my addiction are considered, there will come the conviction that all the benefits it has conferred upon humanity will not atone for the sin it is guilty of towards a single individual who is its helpless slave.

Not only do we once again see the drug considered as an animate agent, capable of innocence and guilt, but we see also the astonishing egotism promoted by De Quincey's legacy. Let a million people agonize after operations, that I might not succumb to weakness!

Needless to say, withdrawal is so painful as to be impossible:

> During the subjection I fought nine times three hundred and sixty-five days against the diabolic master. Again and again the adversary seemed nearly overcome, the daily quantity having been reduced to a minimum, while in one titanic contest there was complete victory for five days; not one drop having entered the mouth in that time. At the end of these one hundred and twenty hours I was in a most deplorable condition. The entire surface of the body was pricked by invisible needles. If one who has felt the painful sensation of a single one will multiply that by ten million, he may dimly grasp the intensity of that form of suffering.... Every joint of the body was racked with consuming fire.... Thus tortured by bodily inquisitorial demons, crazed by wild darting nerves, and devoured by apprehension of shapeless death, I held out my hand and, placing the poisoned chalice to my lips, soon subsided into physical quiet and mental torpor.

Demons, inquisitors, torture, the rack: there is a pattern in the hyperbole. The reader of opiate literature soon recognizes the metaphors. Cobbe repeats:

> The poppy never suffers a man to get out of its spell for a single moment. To be suddenly snatched away from it is to meet certain death or insanity.

The contradiction here is so obvious that it hardly needs pointing out: for by the time he writes, Cobbe is no longer taking opiates in any form. All the apparatus of slavery, chains and demoniac possession has not been sufficient to prevent him from abandoning the drug. But the metaphor, like the grin of the Cheshire cat, is left behind, and leaves (as it is intended to leave) an indelible impression on the mind of the reader, who will subsequently use it himself—and thus it enters popular terminology and then mythology.

In 1907, Léon Daudet, the son of Alphonse, and himself a doctor, published a novel entitled *La Lutte* (The Struggle), and subtitled *A Novel of a Cure*. The protagonist, a doctor, starts to take morphine for his tuberculosis, and then becomes addicted. He enters a clinic in Germany, where he undergoes withdrawal by very rapid reduction of his dosage.

> The night dragged on without advancing, like a drunkard lying in a ditch. I replied to the enquiries of my nurse only by groans. During the succession of dreams and sudden awakenings which followed, I seemed often to feel his bearded head as he listened to my chest. We were no doubt entering that dangerous zone sown with reefs and shipwrecks, which comes thirty hours after almost total abstinence. The memories of my studies and reading came back to me in little scraps, with titles in English and German: *The Opium Habit and Its Treatment ... Pathologie der Morphiumsucht.* I perceived a field of poppies in full light, ready for harvest, then rotten and unusable. Like a drowning man clutching a branch, I held on to the memory of she whom I loved. She ran the whole length of my torture with the speed of a will-o'-the-wisp, but I couldn't see her blurred features clearly ... the idea of escape occurred to the wounded, murdered prisoner.... In the interval between two periods of choking, I asked [Uberthurm, the doctor] "Why don't you let me die instead of . . ." He knew the rest of the sentence .... I looked for a means of suicide. There was still a glass on my table. I could seize it, break it between my teeth, and swallow the fragments before Uberthurm or Fritz [the nurse] could stop me. Not very encouraging to those who want to give up.

Unfortunately, exaggeration of the horrors of withdrawal were not confined at the time to literary types. Doctors themselves, taking their patients' sufferings at their word, repeated them. There was thus a dialectic set up between literary and medical convention. Even Dr. Chambard, the French psychiatrist of the late nineteenth century, whose prose was so lucid, was guilty. Here is his description of how a patient might be withdrawn suddenly from opiates, with all the necessary precautions:

> Abrupt withdrawal necessitates the admission of the addict to an asylum or an institution specializing in drug addiction, but also special methods of surveillance within these institutions.... As soon as he is admitted, the patient takes a bath while his clothes and belongings are minutely searched for the reserves of morphine

that might be hidden in them. He is then placed in a special section of the establishment, in which he will have no contact not only with the other patients, but with the staff who deal with them. His room, whose door is carefully sealed and whose windows are arranged so that there is no possibility of escape, or suicidal jumping, or communication with other people, is very simply furnished with a bed fixed to the wall, a night table, and a chaise longue, without any object that can be displaced, broken and used as a weapon during his crises of agitation. Heating is provided by a hidden stove and he is provided with light by a lamp ... beyond his reach. A bathroom is prepared in the immediate vicinity of this room and the section for drug addicts has a lounge where those who have come through the stormy period of withdrawal may meet and overcome by means of company and various games the inevitable suffering caused by the treatment and the boredom of imprisonment.... It is known that all drug addicts who ask to be interned in a hospital, an asylum or nursing home, to cure his habit definitively, treats himself, before the beginning of his treatment and abstinence, to a de luxe dose: he makes his farewell to his life as a drug addict like a man quitting his life as a bon viveur. The first twenty-four hours are generally calm; but after ... one sees develop a state of growing irritation which can become a state of real mania; and this fact is so regular that one can say that, if it fails to arise, the patient has succeed in one of the ruses in which such patients are so expert. It is then necessary to watch over the patient, and steel one's heart against all his supplications and threats, remove from him anything that could serve as a weapon, stop all possible attempts at escape and even suicide, thwart all the ruses that he employs to obtain a clandestine supply of morphine ...

Once this stage is over, boredom—says Chambard—is the main enemy of the drug addict. It induces him to resume his habit. But clearly for Chambard (an excellent writer, far better than De Quincey), withdrawal is something terrible.

Another writer who straddled medicine and literature, Mikhail Bulgakov, wrote a series of medical stories, one of which was entitled "Morphine." In it, a country doctor has addicted himself to morphine. He describes the pains of withdrawal thus, ironically contrasting what he experiences with a textbook of medicine description of withdrawal as "a morbid anxiety, a depressed nervous condition, irritability":

> "Depressed condition" indeed! Having suffered from this appalling malady, I hereby enjoin all doctors to be more compassionate towards their patients. What overtakes the addict deprived of morphine for a mere hour or two is not "a depressed condition": it is slow death. Air is insubstantial, gulping it down is useless ... there is not a cell in one's body that does not crave ... But crave what? This is something that defies analysis and explanation. In short, the individual ceases to exist: he is eliminated. The body which moves, agonizes and suffers is a corpse. It wants nothing, can think of nothing but morphine. The feeling must be something like that of a man buried alive, clawing at the skin on his chest in the effort to catch the last bubbles of air in his coffin, or of a heretic at the stake, groaning and writhing as the first tongues of flame lick at his feet.
>
> Death. A dry, slow death. That is what lurks behind that clinical, academic phrase "a depressed condition."

Though Bulgakov is writing fiction, there is nothing in the story to suggest that he does not accept this account as the literal truth: indeed, the dramatic force of the story depends upon it being the literal truth, and the reason why the doctor cannot give up the drug and finally commits suicide. In a sense, De Quincey may be said to have killed him (Bulkgakov's stories were, of course, based on actual cases).

Medical exaggeration of the severity of withdrawal continued long after Chambard and Bulgakov, and indeed until the present day, fed by popular images of the condition. Most of the junior doctors in my hospital are still of the opinion that it is something terrible, far worse than withdrawal from alcohol. Here is a description written by a doctor in 1958, and quoted in a book for the general public published by Penguin Books for the mass market in 1964, just as the drug culture was expanding to become not aberrant but the supposed vanguard of a superior, kindlier civilization:

> "Withdrawal sickness" in one with well-developed physical dependence on opiates is a shattering experience and even a physician accustomed to the sight of suffering finds it an ordeal to watch the

agonies of patients in this condition ... the addict begins to enter
the lower depths of his personal hell.... So extreme are the con-
tractions of the intestines that the surface of the abdomen appears
corrugated and knotted as if a tangle of snakes were fighting
beneath the skin.... Thirty-six hours after his last dose of the drug
the addict presents a truly dreadful spectacle.... His whole body
is shaken by twitchings.... Filthy, unshaven, dishevelled, befouled
with his own vomit and faeces, the addict at this stage presents an
almost subhuman appearance ... His weakness may become so
great that he literally cannot raise his head. No wonder many
physicians fear for the very lives of their patients.

While withdrawal from opiates alone is now acknowledged not
to cause hallucinations, it appears that listening to the complaints
of patients can induce hallucinations in physicians. It must be
acknowledged that, since expectations in this instance (including
those of third parties such as doctors) deeply affect and almost
determine symptoms, compassionate and empathic physicians
actually cause the suffering with which they sympathize and
empathize. In the above case, however, the sympathy seems to be
tinged with relish for the extreme and extravagantly disgusting
nature of the symptoms. La Rochefoucauld said that there is in
the misfortune of our friends something not entirely unpleasing;
and no doubt a mildly sadistic doctor can satisfy his illicit desires
while appearing compassionate by dwelling on the sufferings of
others, real or supposed.

But let us return briefly to the errors, or lies, of laymen.
Cocteau wrote, "Nothing better illustrates the drama of disin-
toxication than those speeded up films which show the grimaces,
the gestures, the contortions of the vegetable kingdom." Drama,
drama, drama, all is drama. The ego speaks louder than words.

In *The Diary of a Drug Fiend,* by Aleister Crowley, the pains
of withdrawal from heroin are described. This is the diary of Sir
Peter's lover, Lou Pendragon:

We lie about and look at each other; but we can't touch, the skin
is too painful ... we can't do anything .... I can't remember the
date .... I don't even know what year it is.... The light of day is
torture. Every sense is the instrument of the most devilish pain.
There is no flesh on our bones. This perpetual craving for H! Our

> minds are utterly empty of everything else.... It is like vitriol being thrown in one's face. We have no expression of our own. We cannot think.... His mind has gone back to infancy. He thought I was his Mother.... He might shoot me in a mad fit.... He talks about a gang of hypnotists that have got hold of him, and put evil thoughts in his mind.... We are living in an eternity of damnation.... Every action is a separate agony rising to a climax that never comes.... I am in a perpetual state of pain. Everything is equally anguish.... The medical books say that if one didn't die outright from abstention ... But I am so young to die!

This is almost as bad as Coleridge.

Nelson Algren's novel *The Man with the Golden Arm* was published in 1959. The blurb of the first edition says that Algren "is the eloquent and compassionate voice for the meek and the lowly, the lost and the damned of this earth, enchained by poverty, frustration and despair." One of the chief characters in the novel, Frankie Machine, is "as tough as any of the regulars at Schwiefka's [gambling joint], but he wasn't tough enough to throw the thirty-five pound monkey that rode his back—which was his way of saying that he couldn't stay too long away from the dope needle." In other words, he is enchained by something impossible to escape.

One reason for this, of course, is the withdrawal effects of heroin. After learning about "the image of one hooked so helplessly on morphine that there would be no getting the monkey off without another's help," we learn that:

> By the time Frankie got inside the room he was so weak Louie had to help him in the army cot beside the oil stove. He lay on his back with one arm flung across his eyes as if in shame; and his lips were blue with cold. The pain had hit him with an icy fist in the groin's very pit, momentarily tapering off to a single probing finger touching the genitals to get the maximum of pain. He tried twisting to get away from the fist: the finger was worse than the fist. His throat was so dry that, though he spoke, the lips moved and made no sound.

Two hundred pages later, things have not improved much. Frankie is withdrawing again, but prepares a dose to obviate his suffering:

Frankie sucked the air out of the medicine dropper, then held a match to the morphine in the tiny glass tube. But his hand shook so that he couldn't steady the flame ... and lay back with the one bared arm upflung and the light overhead making hollows of anguish under his eyes. His whole forehead glistened whitely with sweat and the throat so stretched with suffering that it shone bloodlessly.

A dead man's throat.

Who can blame him if he takes to the needle yet again? Alexander Trocchi's book, published a year later, loses no time in letting us know of the horrors of withdrawal:

> Sometimes I think of all those ignorant cops, all those ignorant judges, all those ignorant bastard people committing bloody murder like they blow their noses! ... anyone with a beard ... will be dealt with cold turkey until they take him before a judge and then, because it can't stand, being bestial, scarcely human, the quivering, blubbering, vomiting mass is given half a grain of morphine ten minutes before he is arraigned so they won't have to take him in on a stretcher and run the risk of some irresponsible goon sending for a doctor!

Quivering, blubbering, vomiting masses; stretchers; death: how dreadful! It is almost enough to make you forget that, in the words of the Dutch textbook:

> [Withdrawal from opiates is] time-limited ... and not life-threatening, thus can be easily controlled by reassurance, personal attention and general nursing care without the need for any pharmacotherapy.

In the introduction to *Naked Lunch,* in the first British edition of 1964, Burroughs wrote:

> I awoke from the Sickness at the age of forty-five.... Most survivors do not remember the delirium in detail. I apparently took detailed notes on sickness and delirium. I have no precise memory of writing the notes ...

There is no delirium in withdrawal from opiates and Burroughs was a liar. He was a complete psychopathic scoundrel for whom the truth, let alone the welfare of others, meant nothing. But he has been believed, as if, like the young George Washington, he could not tell a lie, by the gullible and the uncritical.

The literary tradition continues up to the present day: who can say that tradition is dead? In 1993, another Scottish novelist, called Irvine Welsh, published a book called *Trainspotting*. It is mostly written in broad Scots dialect, not altogether easy to read, yet the book has sold millions and was made into a film. Taken as utterly authentic, because deeply repellent, the book soon has much to say on the question of withdrawal:

> He wis takin nae notice though. Ah stoaped harassing him, knowing this ah wis jist wastin ma energy. His silent suffering through withdrawal now seemed so intense that thir wis nae way that ah could add, even incrementally, tae his misery.

Then the protagonist decides to withdraw from heroin. As befits so terrible an experience to come, he makes elaborate plans:

> Third time lucky. It wis like Sick boy telt us: you've got tae know what it's like tae try tae come off it before ye can actually dae it. You can only learn through failure, and what ye learn is the importance ay preparation.... Anywey, this time ah've prepared. A month's rent in advance oan this big, bare room overlooking the Links. Too many bastards ken ma Montgomery Street address.... Partin with that poppy wis the hardest bit. The easiest wis ma last shot, taken in ma left airm this morning. Ah needed something tae keep us gaun during this period ay intense preparation. Then ah wis off like a rocket ... whizzing though ma shopping list.
>
> Ten tins ay Heinz tomato soup, eight tins ay mushroom soup (all to be consumed cold), one large tub ay vanilla ice-cream (which will melt and be drunk), two boatils ay Milk of Magnesia, one boatil of paracetemol, one packet ay Rinstead mouth pastilles, one boatil ay multivits, five litres ay mineral water, twelve Lucozade isotonic drinks and some magazines: soft porn, *Viz, Scottish Football Today, The Punter,* etc. The most important item hus already been procured from a visit tae the parental home; ma Ma's bottle ay valium, removed from her bathroom cabinet.... It's going tae be a hard week.

Preparations continue:

> Ah've goat three brown plastic buckets, half-filled wi a mixture
> ay disinfectant and water for ma shite, puke and pish. Ah line up
> ma tins ay soup, juice and ma medicines within easy reach ay ma
> makeshift bed.

It isn't long, of course, before terrible suffering sets in:

> Ay took ma last shot in order tae get us through the horrors ay
> the shopping trip. Ma final score will be used tae help us sleep,
> and ease us oaf the skag. Ah'll try to take it in small, measured
> doses. Ah need some quickly. The great decline is setting in. It
> starts as it generally does, with a slight nausea in the pit ay ma
> stomach and an irrational panic attack. As soon as ah become
> aware ay the sickness gripping me, it effortlessly moves from the
> uncomfortable to the unbearable.

One may wonder, of course, about the resilience of a man who
cannot face the "horrors" of a little shopping that would take
about fifteen minutes to complete without an injection of heroin,
and it is clear that he is experiencing withdrawal before he could
possibly be withdrawing. Unbearability is like the irresistibility
of irresistible impulses. Irresistible or unresisted? Unbearable or
not borne?

Things, of course, get worse:

> A toothache starts tae spread frae ma teeth intae ma jaws and ma
> eye sockets, and aw through ma bones in a miserable, implacable,
> debilitating throb. The auld sweats arrive on cue, and lets no for-
> get the shivers, covering ma back like a thin layer ay autumn frost
> on a car roof.

So terrible is all this that his resolution falters—within a very
short time, so it seems. The suffering must be great indeed.

> No way can ah crash oot and face the music yet.

He gives up and decides to find some heroin:

> The only thing ah kin move for is smack.

The reader is left with the impression of a harrowing experience
which no one could be blamed for avoiding. That an ability to

move only in order to obtain heroin cannot be purely physiological in nature is lost in all the effluvia of withdrawal.

I accidentally discovered a general reader's response to the
withdrawal scene in *Trainspotting* when I went to a local post
office to pick up a parcel. I was carrying the book with me, having decided, somewhat reluctantly, to read it for the purposes of
writing this chapter. A man behind the counter at the post office
saw that I had the book with me and said enthusiastically, "That's
a very good book, isn't it."

"No," I replied, "it's a very bad book."

He looked amazed: how could anyone not think *Trainspotting* was a very good book?

"What do you mean?" he asked.

"I mean it is an extremely vulgar book and much of it is
untruthful."

"Untruthful?"

"About heroin withdrawal. It isn't at all like that."

"You mean it's far worse than he says?"

That it might not be as bad was something completely
beyond the range of possibilities entertained by his mind.

It is, of course, never too young to indoctrinate children
with the theology of De Quincey's true church. A novel for
teenagers entitled *Junk* was published in Britain in 1996, became
a best-seller and was duly awarded the country's premier prize
for novels for adolescents. The novel is recounted through the
eyes of several characters, and concerns mainly a group of young
adolescents who have run away from home because of various
forms of abuse they suffered there. Some of them addict themselves to heroin, and it is from this addiction that the book derives
its principal interest, fame, and notoriety. There had been plenty
of books about opiates and heroin before, but none for readers
so young. It will by now come as no great surprise to the reader
to learn that the author, Melvin Burgess, accepts and promotes
the view that withdrawal from heroin is a truly terrible experience, and that, once a person has become addicted, he needs professional help to stop taking the drug. At the end of the book,
one of the addicts called Tar says:

> I went to see the doctor and told him about it [his craving for
> heroin after he had stopped taking it for a while], but he wouldn't
> give me any methadone because I hadn't done any junk. So I went
> away and had a think about it. I knew I wasn't going to make it
> without help. The next day I went back and told him I'd lied, I
> had done some ... so I told a few fibs, told him it was just the
> other week when in fact it was over two months back. But it
> worked. I got my script. All in a good cause, getting me clean
> again.

The effect of this is not only to normalize and legitimize drug-
taker's jargon ("I hadn't done any junk"), but to teach a very
important lesson: that self-inflicted problems can be solved only
with professional or technical assistance, and not by the exercise
of will. This is an old lesson, but that has repeatedly to be learned,
in each successive generation. A medical textbook of 1913, *The
Narcotic Drug Diseases and Allied Ailments* by Dr. George Pettey,
states, "The exercise of the will alone is sufficient to interrupt and
suspend any course of conduct arising entirely from force of habit.
That is not true of narcotic disease; therefore, it is not a mere
habit and should not be spoken of as such."

Earlier in the book, Tar had detoxified in a rehabilitiation
unit:

> Then came the bad bit—withdrawal. Cold turkey. I never had it
> so bad. I suppose the truth is I always had a little bit here and there
> to help me through.... It was awful. I nearly cracked. I would
> have done, if I was on my own.

Fortunately, there were counsellors and other addicts, who had
had the same terrible experience, to help him through. "They're
not full of the bullshit you normally get from people who've never
had the problem." Yes, only addicts have true knowledge: not De
Quincey, therefore, but Tar, and by implication every addict, is
the infallible pope of his own church.

Another of the protagonists in the book, also a heroin addict,
is a young girl called Gemma. Together with Tar and other addict
friends, they take a break in the countryside in an earlier attempt
to withdraw. She says:

I'd tried to give up about half a dozen times, but I'd never been scared before. I mean, you gotta take risks, we'd all been scared about ODing, or about getting stuck forever on junk, or about buggering up our veins, that sort of stuff. But that's just normal. This time was different, and I knew I was a junkie this time because, what's a junkie scared of? Not Aids, not overdosing, like you might think. We were scared because there might be no more smack at the other end. . . . It was the first time I knew I couldn't get by without it.

This, of course, is intended to be entirely plausible: withdrawal is worse than both lingering disease and death itself. It seems to me unlikely that adolescents would read that passage very critically. It implies, and is intended to imply, that withdrawal from opiates is a fate worse than death, which therefore explains why people continue to take them, and why medical assistance is so imperatively necessary for addicts if they are to give up.

You are never too young to be wilfully and woefully misled. I do not expect the balefully misleading literary tradition to die out in the very near future.

INDEX